PRAISE FOR THE GREATEST BLESSING

"Very few people willingly make the choice to serve as a caregiver, but many will find themselves in this role at some point. *The Greatest Blessing* isn't a guidebook, yet it beautifully captures the full range of emotions, burdens, and yes, blessings of caregiving. Most importantly, it shows us what we're capable of enduring in the name of love."

-JAMES H. DOUGLAS
Former governor of Vermont and current executive in residence at Middlebury College

"We need these stories to remind us that the love we share with our families is what gives us the strength, courage, perseverance and everything else we need to grow from adversity and even find gratitude for it."

-ARON LEE RALSTON
New York Times **bestselling author and subject of the Oscar-nominated film** *127 Hours*

"None of us knows what life has in store for us. How would we react when a loved one is stricken, and we're suddenly thrust into the role of caregiver? This book supplies example after example of how trial and tragedy can offer an opening for grace and growth. Each account is a blessing in its own right, a reminder that no matter how hard the road ahead, someone else has traveled it and come through transformed. Listen to this testimony and be inspired, comforted, and reassured."

-ALEXANDER WOLFF
New York Times **bestselling author and award-winning** *Sports Illustrated* **writer**

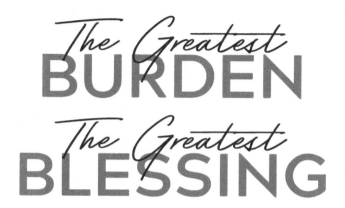

The Greatest
BURDEN
The Greatest
BLESSING

Compliments of

Watertown
—— **Savings Bank** ——

Best Wishes

The Greatest BURDEN
The Greatest BLESSING

Caregiving stories of
hope, humility, and love.

Mark J. Resnick
Alan E. Rubel
Michael D. Tenaglia

The conversations, events, and locales in the book all come from the authors' recollections, though they are not written to represent word-for-word transcripts. Rather, they are retold in a way that evokes the feeling and meaning of what was said, and, in all instances, the essence of the dialogue is accurate.

Although every effort was made to ensure that the information in this book was correct at press time, the authors and publisher do not assume or hereby disclaim any liability caused by errors or omissions, whether such errors or omissions result from negligence, accident, or any other cause.

The content and resources in this book are provided for informational purposes only and should not be used to replace the specialized training and professional judgement of a health care or mental health care professional.

First paperback edition August 2023

Covers designed by Murphy Rae
Cover photo by Kim Johnson
Edited by Shaina Clingempeel
Formatting by Alejandro Martin

ISBN 979-8-9857494-4-1 (paperback)
ISBN 979-8-9857494-5-8 (ebook)
ISBN 979-8-9857494-6-5 (hardcover)
ISBN 979-8-9857494-7-2 (audio)

Published by Mark J. Resnick Media
www.markjresnick.com
www.caregivingguys.com

"The battle rages on . . .
It's been ten years since Lynda was diagnosed with cancer.
Now, it feels like we're on a rowboat heading straight for Niagara Falls.
Lynda's medical teams are on the banks of the river, throwing us lifelines,
but the water is getting faster and rougher. It's becoming harder to stay
afloat, but we hang on to whatever lines are thrown our way."

—Michael Tenaglia, co-author

This book is dedicated to the millions of personal
caregivers—the invisible patients—for your unending
love and commitment to your care recipient(s).

We see you.

TABLE OF CONTENTS

About the Cover image:

Kim Johnson is a self-taught photographer based out of Milton, DE. He finds inspiration from the vastly different and beautiful beaches, parks, farms, wildlife, and landscapes of Delmarva, DE. To see more of his work, visit Kimjohnsonphotographyde.com, or you can find him on Facebook.

About the Cover design:

In 2015, Murphy Rae downloaded Photoshop on a whim and decided to give design a shot. Since then, she has received her certificate in graphic design from Southern Methodist University and designed hundreds of book covers for a range of authors, from those navigating self-publishing for the first time, to seasoned *USA Today* and *New York Times* best-selling authors. Visit www.murphyrae.com for more information.

About the Editor:

Shaina Clingempeel is an expert editor who lives in New York. After earning her Writing MFA from Sarah Lawrence College, she developed a deep passion for helping people share their stories. As a writer herself, she is especially dedicated and precise. Now she works with new and established writers and guides them in the development of their work, as if it were her own. Visit www.shainaclingempeel.com for more information.

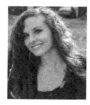

FOREWORD

Rasheda Ali Walsh

By the time I realized my father was famous, I was six or seven years old, and he was diligently working on a world heavyweight boxing title. Later that year, on September 15, 1978, he accomplished that goal by defeating Leon Spinks, and in doing so, he became the first fighter in history to win the World Heavyweight Championship three times.

To the rest of the world, Muhammad Ali was the greatest boxer of all time. During his twenty-one-year boxing career, he was a multiple Golden Glove winner, an Olympic champion, and a three-time world heavyweight champion. Before retiring in 1981, he accumulated a 56–5 record with thirty-seven knockouts.

I always believed he was the greatest, too. But to me, he was simply the greatest friend and father. From a very young age, my siblings and I knew we had to share our dad with the world, but we also knew how much he loved us. He was a loving, generous, caring, and sensitive family man. When we spoke on the phone, he often recorded us; he said it was important to cherish such memories with his children.

As much as my dad loved being Muhammad Ali, he also suffered throughout his personal and professional life. He sacrificed his career, livelihood, and time spent with us to make this world a better place—to stand up for freedom, justice, and equality. I realized how impactful his words and actions were across the globe. Using his fame to spotlight peace, help the poor, and speak up for the voiceless—those were his greatest accomplishments to society.

There were so many times I watched my dad rise, fall, and rise again, both in and out of the boxing ring. The world will never forget his rise to fame in one of the greatest upsets in boxing history. In this historic bout as an underdog against the Heavyweight Champion Sonny Liston, no one would have predicted that it wasn't his most challenging fight—not by a long shot. His toughest fight was against the complicated, progressive, neurocognitive condition known as Parkinson's disease.

Diagnosed with Parkinson's in 1984, he spent the next thirty-two years battling the disease. Although slurred speech was one of my father's most cumbersome and inconvenient symptoms of his condition, he bravely accepted the challenge and continued to lead by example. He motivated and inspired us to serve others, by helping people evolve physically, mentally, and spiritually—and he encouraged others to become the best versions of themselves. I feel his greatest accomplishments were outside of the ring, including his contributions to raising awareness for neurocognitive diseases. It continues to be a privilege and honor to carry on my dad's legacy by advocating on behalf of Parkinson's disease patients and their families.

One day, Daddy and I were having a deep conversation about careers, and I stressed to him how challenging it was breaking into the world of performing arts. My father gave me the best advice under the circumstances, and that was to ignore the obstacles that presented themselves and to continue to pursue my dreams regardless of outside factors that stood in my way. Despite his visible health challenges, my father had no hesitation in offering such advice to me regarding my confidence. I knew immediately that this show of affection had to be the inner workings of someone not only on an elevated spiritual plane but also someone great.

The conversation reminded me that those who have been touched by Parkinson's disease and other neurocognitive conditions are still the same person on the inside. He was still my dad, only he was trapped in a body that didn't always allow him to complete simple tasks that we take for granted. Small gestures like walking, eating, uninterrupted sleep, dressing, and speaking clearly.

I personally feel that God put him on this earth for a reason. My dad always shared with us that everything in life has a purpose which is why I feel he never complained about his condition and continued to help others and never stopped sharing his gifts. At times, it was difficult during the late stages of Parkinson's disease, to walk and talk, but Dad continued to fulfill his purpose on earth: to give to others. Honestly, I think that Parkinson's disease gave my dad a deeper meaning to his life.

Throughout the years of my father's struggles with Parkinson's disease, I pitched in to help his care partners whenever I could. As I discovered fairly quickly, it takes a special, selfless individual to take on the role of Care Partner, and it also requires an incredible amount of patience and the assistance of family, friends, and other support systems. It became the motivation behind my children's book, *I'll Hold Your Hand So You Won't Fall*. In order to help our loved ones, we need to educate ourselves—including children and young people—on the disease and the behaviors associated with it. We want to protect and shield them from watching someone they love suffer, but it's important for them to be a part of the caregiving process, even if their only role is to make someone smile or laugh.

Which brings me to you, the caregiver.

It doesn't matter if you're in the early, middle, or late stages of your caregiving journey—or even if your role has ended. I understand the burdens imposed upon you and your family and will offer some advice based on my experience caring for my dad, as well as witnessing others do the same for their loved ones.

Continue to educate yourself and others about your recipient's condition. Ask for help. Build or join a support group and know and understand your rights as a patient.

Never give up on making your loved one feel special and cherished. Give them as much independence as possible, so long as you're not sacrificing your own health. And understand the importance of having patience and understanding, especially during the challenging times.

Don't forget that you're not alone in this courageous battle. There are others who have walked your path and continue to serve as special heroes to their loved ones every day.

Most importantly, don't ever lose sight of caring for yourself and improving *your* quality of life as well. Life's challenges make it easy to forget about *your* physical, mental, and spiritual well-being during the duties of being an excellent caregiver. Yet without a healthy mind, body, and soul, you may find it that much more difficult to deliver the care you so desire.

Life will undoubtedly throw challenges your way, but one of the most inspiring things I've learned from my father during his fight with Parkinson's disease was learning how to be courageous. He followed the inspirational words of Nelson Mandela, who said, "The greatest glory in living lies not in never falling, but in rising every time we fall."

You're about to read example after example of what it means to be courageous in *The Greatest Burden The Greatest Blessing*. Sometimes it's the care recipient, and sometimes it's the care partner, but the amount of courage, compassion, hope, humility, kindness, and love demonstrated throughout this book is, quite simply, the greatest.

Best of luck on your journey to unconditional love and commitment as a caregiver.

Rasheda Ali Walsh

Rasheda Ali is an internationally known author, speaker, actress, spokesperson and Parkinson's disease advocate. Her book, *I'll Hold Your Hand So You Won't Fall-A Child's Guide to Parkinson's Disease*, was inspired by her children and her father, Muhammad Ali, who suffered more than 30 years from the disease.

As an advocate of stem cell research, Rasheda travels the globe motivating others to make a difference in their communities, raising awareness and funds for neurocognitive disorders as well as promoting love and inclusion through the Muhammad Ali Center. As a member of the Screen Actors Guild and the American Federation of Television and Radio Artists, Rasheda served as writer, casting director and host for her own celebrity talk show in Las Vegas. Most recently, Rasheda was cast in a film which is currently streaming nationwide on Tubi.

FOREWORD

Brett Miller

Joining the United States Army four days after graduating high school to become a combat medic was the best decision of my life. By the time I graduated from boot camp at age eighteen, I was physically and mentally fit, proud, and the sharpest I'd ever been. It was the beginning of the rest of my life—I could be anything I wanted to be and accomplish anything I was willing to work for.

Keep running towards your dreams, they said.

Six years later, I was deployed to Bosnia to serve under the European Command Specials Operations Teams. The conflict between the Serbs and Croatians had officially ended in 1995 with the signing of the Dayton Agreement, but our peacekeeping and protection role was vital to the survival of hundreds of thousands of people left to deal with the war's utter devastation.

We pulled people out of their broken homes and led them to camps, where they could then get safely to other countries to triage them. Thousands of buried mines blew up innocent civilians, and I treated them in the streets or fields, always under some very archaic medical conditions. Despite our NATO Humanitarian effort, we encountered many situations under gunfire that could've become ransom, torture, or execution situations. I wasn't running toward my dreams—I was running to safety and helping others do the same.

I survived the trenches of Bosnia but still see the faces of the men, women, and children I cared for who lost limbs from exploded mines. I see refugees torn from their families as a result of one of the worst massacres in history. It was a type of caregiving I wish to never experience again, but caring it was.

After chasing the demons of my past out of my life for good, I was able to finally start chasing my dreams, just like my commanding officers encouraged me to thirty-plus years ago. Writing the foreword to a book on caregiving was never one of those dreams, yet I find myself pinching myself anyway. It is, I would say, one of the greatest blessings.

What you're about to read—a collection of the most inspirational and moving accounts of caregiving from people far braver and more resilient than I ever was—will be something you will never forget.

Only for good reasons.

Reflecting on my own caregiving journey—not only in Bosnia but with my diabetic brother and my father and his nine heart attacks—I can appreciate the true hope and beautiful silver linings so thoughtfully articulated in this book. Yes, you will enter the trenches—the mental and physical warfare of caregiving—but somehow will come out of the muck and mire with more love, patience, and compassion for others.

In *The Greatest Burden The Greatest Blessing*, you will come to understand the universal power and gift of caring for a loved one, as well as how caregivers transcend grief and loss. Even when they reached a breaking point, these caregivers displayed unimaginable strength to carry on, to endure. Some never felt more alive, others never more broken. But all of the writers implicitly express that no one should go on this journey alone.

Through their combined years and experience in caregiving, community involvement, and writing, the three gentlemen leading the charge have masterfully created a collection of stories that are profoundly inspirational. Most will pick up this book because of the title alone: *The Greatest Burden The Greatest Blessing*. Not only does it perfectly encapsulate what you're about to read, but it justifies my life path—and the path of millions of others who provide care, coaching, and guidance to those who need it most.

Get ready to witness the journeys of incredible, everyday heroes who have come out, or are currently enthralled, in the battle that is caregiving.

You will notice that there are no white flags present within the forthcoming pages. Only recognition of the blessings, and sometimes spiritual awakenings, which comes from selfless acts of love. You will also notice the acute attention to details, the insatiable quest for knowledge and understanding, the intangible ingredients used to cope and thrive—and the number of times these caregivers bent but never broke.

The Greatest Burden The Greatest Blessing is a reminder that we are exactly where we need to be when the call to be a caregiver comes. It's a book of everyday heroes. It's a book about hope, true grit, and deep love.

It's a book that reminds us that no matter how difficult, draining, and dark caring for a loved one can be, we must never stop running toward our dreams. Because the recipients of our care—our loved ones—would never want us to stop moving forward.

Brett Miller

Brett Miller is the founder and owner of 110 Fitness in Rockland, Massachusetts, the largest wellness center in the world for individuals with Parkinson's disease. A licensed physical therapist with 27 years of experience, he is a former U.S. Army veteran and author of the book, *It's a Beautiful Day to Save Lives: A Medic's Journey to His Destiny*, available on Amazon.

Brett serves as the co-chair for the Massachusetts Parkinson's Registry as well as a Commissioner on the Massachusetts State Athletic Commission. He also serves as an ambassador for the Michael J. Fox Foundation for Parkinson's Research and the Davis Phinney Foundation. To connect with Brett, please visit www.110fitness.org.

INTRODUCTION

Nothing can prepare you for the call. It might rouse you from a deep sleep in the middle of the night or come gradually over a few weeks, months, or years. Chances are, it will come when you least expect it. You will almost certainly be unprepared, but your decision to answer it—whether by choice or circumstance—will change lives. And not just the care recipients.

For us, it was Alzheimer's and cancer. Long, arduous, gut-wrenching battles against two terrible afflictions. It was, quite simply, the greatest burden of our lives.

The Greatest Burden The Greatest Blessing is a unique collection of stories from fifty caregivers, united not by anger, grief, exhaustion, or despair—but in knowing what they were capable of enduring in the name of love. Despite the enormous burdens placed upon them, most experienced beautiful, heartfelt, and genuine blessings. The three of us certainly have.

Yet unlike most caregiving books, this one doesn't go deep on one disease or perspective; rather, it features bite-sized chapters on a wide range of caregiving experiences. Rooted in hope, humility, and love, the stories you are about to read were written by neighbors, coworkers, parents, siblings, and spouses alike. Each one answered the call to be a caregiver; each mustered the strength and courage to share their story.

Remarkable people. Perhaps even heroic. Yet none of them would view themselves in that manner. Nor should they. After all, they answered the call by choice or circumstance, which is another way of saying, "not by choice." That's what Janet Steward (page 175) experienced, and yet the care she provided her mother was divine.

There is no course or manual on how to be a caregiver. Even if you're a paid caregiver or doctor or nurse, when it comes to caring for your own loved ones, the rules, playing field, and playbooks are different—as if written in another language. Some of you work a full day, then come home to manage symptoms, which can change by the hour, as well as administer meds, clean up messes, navigate the health care and insurance system, communicate with family, deal with doctors, and advocate for the right care, even when you're not sure what that means. Or you catch up with your loved one and try to put a smile on their face. Or you sit in silence, which can be equally meaningful.

Because there's a critical shortage of paid professional caregivers and skilled nurses, the burdens placed upon the personal caregiver become greater and the level of stress more poignant. It's not hyperbolic to say that caregiving might kill you. Not the recipient of your care, the one with the disease or injury. We're talking about you—the caregiver.

I know the words, *it might just kill you,* are not the same as "She has two weeks to two months to live," like Sara Robinson heard, or when Matt Perrin was told, "Your Mom has Alzheimer's." And it's certainly not the same as hearing, "We think you have ALS," as Reverend Jennifer Durant, a wife and mother of two children, did in 2012.

We get it, but would be remiss to warn you otherwise, for there may be no greater burden in life than that of caregiving.

Nicole Bell was the caregiver for her husband, who had early-onset Alzheimer's. Her story, found on page 269, talks about the post-caregiving experience. Yet in her memoir, *What Lurks in the Woods: Struggle and Hope in the Midst of Chronic Illness,* she wrote:

"Like a guided missile, [Shannon] unearthed my deepest torment. I was so freaking tired of being strong. I had to be strong for the kids, making them feel like everything was okay and normal. I had to be strong at work, leading everyone through each technical hurdle and challenge. I had to be strong to keep the house running, learning new things I'd never done before. And I had to be strong for the one person I relied upon. The person who gave me strength and grounded me in everything I did. But now, that person was slowly becoming more of a burden. He dragged me down into depths I'd never been before. So I was forced to become stronger in order to survive. But I was so tired, tired of being strong."

Diana Pierce has served patients and their caregivers for more than forty years. On page 247, she wrote:

"The role of caregiving is usually one of benevolent intentions and actions. Offering care to those in need is as old as humanity. Receiving care is often a humbling and at times difficult experience. The offering and receiving of care can be one of the most loving and grace-filled acts between humans. It can also be overwhelming, soul-deep fatiguing, frustrating, and all-consuming of one's time, energy, and finances."

Cole was diagnosed with neuroblastoma cancer at age six. The odds of his survival were about thirty-five percent. His dad, Tony Stoddard, wrote on page 71:

"Multiple surgeries, radiation treatments, and rounds of chemotherapy began—it tore my soul to bits to watch my son suffer so deeply. My wife was so incredibly strong throughout the year and a half that Cole battled cancer. She somehow found the strength to stay organized each day, scheduling appointments, keeping track of Cole's medications and procedures, and making sure that Troy and Tara lived each day as normally as possible. Honestly, I don't know how she did it. I found that my role as a caretaker during this horrific situation was to simply be a silly dad, focused on helping my kids to smile and laugh, playing with them, and fighting to have Cole at home as much as possible to be with the ones he loved."

The caregiving burden has no floor or ceiling, and yet Sara, Matt, Nicole, Diana, and Tony—and the more than forty other contributors in *The Greatest Burden The Greatest Blessing*—not only found a way to move forward but did so with hope, humility, and love.

If you're currently serving as a caregiver, please know that no matter how large or small your caregiving role is, you make a difference each and every day you show up for your loved one. As the caregiver, you may feel like the invisible patient most of the time, as Jamie Jacobs talks about in her story (page 251), but we see you. Know that you are not alone. Know that you are appreciated. And know that you are loved.

If you've already taken up the gauntlet of caregiving, you have our eternal respect and gratitude. No matter the tragedy or tribulations faced, *you answered the call.* Either way, you're not an angel or a hero; you're simply a caregiver who has experienced one of life's greatest burdens and greatest blessings. Hopefully, you have found the peace and tranquility you deserve for your compassion, commitment, and love for a spouse, significant other, parent, sibling, child, friend, or family member.

In the back of the book, you will find a resources section. Consider it a starting point for your caregiving journey. But no matter what stage of caregiving you're at, we can't emphasize this point enough: ask for help. Caregiving isn't something you want or can afford to do on your own. It's a lesson most of us learned the hard way.

If you find this book helpful, please share it with family and friends. If you'd like to share your caregiving story for future books, visit our website, www.caregivingguys.com.

With gratitude,
Mark, Alan, and Michael

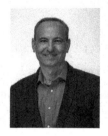 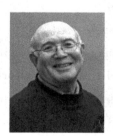 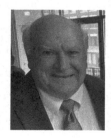

BEAMING WITH BLESSINGS

by Ed Devitt

with Mark J. Resnick

On June 12, 1997, I was recognized as Father of the Year by All Metro Health Care, a health care services agency. It was an honor I wish I never received, not because it wasn't deserved, but because of the circumstances that made me eligible for the award in the first place.

Almost exactly four years prior, on June 23, 1994, my nineteen-year-old daughter, Kelly, and a friend were driving on a rural road in Burlington, Vermont. Both were students at the University of Vermont. The girls were on their way to a nearby park. Under normal circumstances, they would have driven right up to a locked gate, but on this night, the gate swung out into the center of the roadway just as they were entering. The results were devastating.

The fourteen-foot long, 280-pound gate, painted dark brown and difficult to see, crashed through the passenger side front windshield like a spear, smashing into the side of Kelly's head. When her friend tried to maneuver the car away from the gate, it caused a second impact on Kelly's head. The impact was so severe that some of Kelly's brain matter splattered onto her friend, and there was a gaping hole on one side of her head.

When emergency personnel arrived at the scene, one of them said, "Don't hurry; it's a decapitation." She was assumed dead at the time of the accident. Fortunately, one of the firemen had the sense to check her pulse. It was weak, but she had one. He started yelling at Kelly, urging her to fight for her life. And fight she did.

It was 3:00 a.m. when I got the call from her friend's mom.

"The doctors at Fletcher Allen Hospital are waiting for your call. God bless you, Mr. Devitt."

Those are not the words you want to hear. I called the hospital and spoke to the emergency room. "How fast can you get here?" the woman on the phone asked. "I'm not sure she will make it through the night."

When Kelly arrived at the hospital, her blood pressure was thirty-two over zero. They were cutting her clothes off in the parking lot, prepping for surgery. They were putting towels on her bleeding head, but they were immediately soaked through with blood.

Rather than driving or waiting for a commercial flight, I chartered a plane at Westchester Airport. I was at Fletcher Allen two hours later, but upon arrival, they told me I couldn't see her yet. I went to a friend's house, and shortly after arriving, they called the house to get my permission to operate.

Dr. Bednar and his team took more of her skull out to relieve pressure. They also removed bone fragments and her right temporal lobe.

"It's a wait-and-see situation," the doctor told me. Then they induced Kelly into a coma.

***

My daughter was an accomplished gymnast. In 1992, she was a New York State gymnastics champion. She was attending UVM on a full gymnastics scholarship and was planning to become a schoolteacher. In her first year at UVM, she was the ECAC Athlete of the Week for her very first two meets and qualified for the NCAA Regionals that year (the first gymnast in school history to do so).

I'm not sharing this information to brag, but to give you some context for her mental and physical shape prior to the accident. Kelly was an elite athlete—which I believe is the only reason she is alive today.

My mental state prior to Kelly's accident was not so elite. I was out of work and going through a divorce. Both my kids were in college, and I lived by myself. To keep busy, I volunteered at the local Children's Hospital, and believe it or not, I was assigned to hang out with a twelve-year-old kid with a brain injury. We played cards or tossed a ball around. Being around kids with brain injuries was uplifting and sad at the same time. I really felt for these kids.

Two weeks later, I got the call about Kelly's accident—a traumatic brain injury. What are the odds? My experience at Children's Hospital gave me a limited view of the caregiving burden for parents, but it did not prepare me for the emotional and physical pain that parents of children with brain injuries endure.

Once Kelly was put into a coma, we had no idea when she would come out of it. This was the hardest part for me—the waiting, the hoping—the trying to stay positive. I stayed with Kelly that first month, and then I had to go back to work. Every Friday after work, I would drive to Vermont to be with her. It was the hardest thing leaving her on Sunday nights. Thankfully, my foreman was top shelf and understood what I was going through. He let me leave work a few hours early on Fridays to get a jump on the commute to Vermont to see Kelly.

After three months at Fletcher Allen, we decided to move Kelly to Helen Hayes Hospital in New York. One, because it was closer to me, and because they had more experience with coma patients. I have to say, the entire staff at Fletcher Allen Hospital in Vermont was excellent, and I'm grateful to every single one of them.

Within a few weeks of her move to Helen Hayes, Kelly did wake up from her coma. It was three and a half months after the accident and initial surgery. She was unable to talk, but she could spell words. Her eyes were dried and irritated, so I took it upon myself to crush up a bag of onions to get her to tear up. That didn't work, and it wasn't the only time I ignored the advice of her medical team.

Her eyes were the least of her problems. For the rest of her life, Kelly would no longer have the use of her legs. She was a quadriplegic. And Kelly was so angry—rightfully so.

"Why me? Why me? This doesn't make sense!"

She cursed up a storm, and each time the nurses touched her, she would scream.

"It's okay," they reassured me. "Every nerve in her body is on fire right now." It took a few months for the bitterness to go away.

Her four-month stay at Helen Hayes was excellent, but there was nothing else they could do for her there. It was time for Kelly to move to a long-term care environment. After lots of research, we picked the Daytar Group Home in Connecticut.

Every night after work, I drove up to see her. I would pick her up out of bed, exercise with her, and push her to get stronger. The staff there didn't like that. They didn't even want me to let her drink water from a straw for fear she might aspirate and get an infection. I did it anyway.

The other residents at Daytar had serious brain or spinal cord injuries. Many were in rough shape, far worse than Kelly. After a year of living there, it became clear to me that this wasn't a long-term solution for Kelly. I didn't believe they pushed Kelly enough to get stronger.

"Your expectations are too high," the doctor said. "What's the big deal about walking?"

"Don't tell me that stuff," I replied. Finally, I told them to go to hell and that I wanted to take her home with me—I wanted to be her caregiver. Everybody was against the idea.

"You don't know what you're doing," everyone said. The physical therapist, the speech therapist, her caregivers. "You don't know what you're getting yourself into."

"Yes. Yes, I do."

The State of Connecticut had to grant permission for me to take care of her so that Social Security would pay for her care. I got permission, and Kelly came home with me in 1996. For the next fifteen years, we had five caregivers and me sharing the load. My days were Friday, Saturday, and Sunday. I did that for fourteen years until my health started to decline.

Fortunately, through a settlement with the State of Vermont, Kelly was awarded a financial compensation in 1999, which allowed her pay for her own care. The gate—the one that was supposed to be locked up at night—went unlocked five times prior to Kelly's accident. They took responsibility for their negligence, and while Kelly wouldn't get her legs back, she was able to pay for her twenty-four-hour medical care.

In 2012, I had ten mini-strokes. My health was failing, but I continued my caregiving schedule until 2021, when I started having some serious headaches. Turns out I had a brain bleed, which filled my skull cavity and put massive pressure on my brain. I finally went to the emergency room. Two more days and I would have been dead.

I'm seventy-six years old now. I still take care of Kelly on Sundays, but the other six days are done by her full-time care team. It's hard to believe it's been thirty years since her accident. When she first came home with me, I didn't know what to feed her. I barely knew how to cook. But it got easier with time, and Kelly was so good with me, so patient.

Mentally, Kelly is nearly 100%, with the exception of some short-term memory loss. But her personality hasn't changed. We have a good time together. We fight, like any other father and daughter, but she's still Kelly.

They warned me that it would be hard, and it was. Even though she's not paralyzed, she has no motor control, so she can't dress herself or use a fork. But she can talk, get around with her wheelchair, and watch the Yankees play on television. She has a life. It may not have been the one she wanted, but we're both so grateful to have each other.

I'll never forget all those tubes coming out of her skull after the accident. Hearing the *beep, beep, beep*—it kept me going. Every day I heard the beeps was a positive sign because she was alive. Then, when she came out of her coma, it was the greatest blessing.

As I told the folks from All Metro Health Care in 1997, "I can only be the father of the year because I have the daughter of the year."

And that's still true today.

Ed Devitt lives in Mount Kisco, New York. While he remains one of Kelly's caregivers, he would not have been able to without the help of some incredible people, including: Kelly's UVM gymnastics coach, Nini, and her husband Tom Anger, very special people; Kevin, Margo, Mary-Jo, and Kevin Jr. Sleeper, a great family; Dr. Martin Bednar and the staff of Fletcher Allen, professional all the way; and Kelly's lawyer, David Cleary, a smart and caring man.

19

SISTERS AGAIN

by Joyce Kahn

Five years ago, my sister, Leslie, underwent a brutal surgery for tongue cancer. The surgeon excised half of her tongue and grafted skin from her arm to fashion the part of the tongue that had been removed. I flew to Maryland to take care of her for six weeks. I went a second time three years later when the cancer had metastasized to her lungs and COVID-19 was starting up. Thank G-d, she survived those cancers and the life-threatening pneumonias she got before the doctors figured out how to treat them.

I was not a long-time caregiver. I was with my sister post-surgery each time, getting her through that difficult period of pain and many adjustments. My sister and I had not been close. Quite frankly, I had been envious of her my whole life. But when she called to tell me her terrifying diagnosis, I told her I would be there to take care of her. Because I could. I was retired and had no pressing responsibilities or obligations. We are family. Family always comes first.

I am not a natural caregiver. I am squeamish and had to overcome my inclination to flee the scene. When family members were allowed to see my sister after the first surgery, I took one look at her, hooked up to so many tubes, and started to faint. Someone had to escort me to the waiting room, where I sat on the floor and elevated my legs until I no longer felt dizzy.

That did not bode well for me as a caregiver.

The first week was exhausting. Les was in pain. I was the gopher. My mom would have said I was no spring chicken. But there I was, sprinting up and down a long flight of stairs between bedroom and kitchen in an effort to prepare foods that my sister would be able to eat. She needed nourishment, but her new tongue made eating and speaking difficult.

I took my cooking role seriously. I cooked from scratch, making and preparing soups and other soft foods that had to be puréed so they felt right to her new mouth. Often, she did not like the texture. It was an uphill battle. Mint chocolate chip ice cream was one item from Trader Joe's that she enjoyed. Unfortunately, I did as well. Along with the foods I had cooked, I also ate more than my share of ice cream. Even with my running up and down stairs, I did not lose an ounce.

I was the point person for dealing with home service providers. I answered the phone and made appointments. I learned to change dressings and administer my sister's meds through her port. The nurse gave me a tutorial on flushing and administering the meds—I was anxious because this was way above my pay grade. I dealt with agencies and support people, was with my sister for all home visits, and drove her to Johns Hopkins for appointments.

I had to drive on multilane highways and then in city neighborhoods. I hate driving in big city traffic. I white-knuckled it. I shopped and cooked and made countless smoothies and soups and healthy meals in an effort to find foods she might like. She didn't like much and didn't eat much. I ran up and down stairs. I kept her company.

I was becoming a caregiver—by no means a natural fit for me.

Before long, I realized I needed to take care of myself, too, or I would burn out. I was always fearful my new caregiver responsibilities would consume me—that I would lose my increasingly fragile identity. My cello teacher in Vermont knew the owner of a cello studio in the area and arranged for me to borrow a cello and bow. I went to the basement, down two flights of stairs to practice, just so I would not bother my sister. It was therapeutic, but because I am more of an artist than a cellist and had the foresight to pack some art supplies, I also painted. During my short breaks, I painted outdoors in the mild climate of a Maryland winter. Painting and practicing the cello helped me maintain my equilibrium and kept me in touch with the activities that were so integral to my identity.

Our prayers were answered, and my sister Les recovered from her cancer. Somehow, I managed to survive in my role as a caregiver as well. It was the hardest thing I've ever had to do in my lifetime.

The upshot? The silver lining? We became close. We became sisters again.

Les' gratitude continues to this day. She recently told me, "You provided comfort, care, and love in a way no one else could." My nephew, who was in law school at the time, says he will never forget what I did for his mother and for him. He, of course, was worried sick about her surviving. I eased his burden. I rose to the tasks because I had to. And I became richer for the experience.

In 2022, I was diagnosed with Large Cell B Lymphoma. After surgery, chemotherapy, and radiation, I am in remission with a good prognosis. While I didn't have a primary caregiver during my treatments, I had a multitude of wonderful people who helped me every step of the way. Some brought meals or drove me to appointments; others checked in on me and put my garden to sleep for the winter. I am grateful for the love and care I received from friends and family, the Care Committee from my synagogue, Facebook friends, and fellow artists.

A TEAM OF CAREGIVERS

by Brenda and Lee Roy

Brenda Roy gave birth to Travis Mathew Roy on April 17, 1975, and for the next twenty years, he lived a life like most. Blond, blue-eyed, and smaller than most boys his age, he spent his first twenty years living in Yarmouth, Maine.

Travis' life was a typical one. He grew up loving sports and getting decent grades throughout his school years. During his first year in high school, he came out of his room one night and said he wanted to talk with Mom and Dad about his goals:

1. Earn an ice hockey scholarship to play at a Division 1 college.
2. Play ice hockey at a professional level, hopefully in the National Hockey League.
3. Not to sell himself short and earn a spot on the U.S. Olympic ice hockey team.

In order to play high level college hockey, Travis worked hard and committed himself to reaching that goal. He transferred from Yarmouth H.S. to North Yarmouth Academy, a private day school nearby. After two years at NYA, he transferred again to Tabor Academy in Marion, MA. "Whatever it takes!"

In the fall of 1995, Travis entered Boston University on a full hockey scholarship. On October 20, wearing number 24 on his back and Boston University on the front, Travis was on the ice, waiting to play in his first collegiate game. The University was recognizing last year's historic season, having captured the 1994–1995 Hockey East and NCAA Championships, along with the locally prestigious Boston Beanpot Tournament. *Travis had made it.* He had achieved goal #1.

Eleven seconds into his first shift, however, Travis' world ended abruptly. Falling forward while checking a player from North Dakota University, he struck his head against the dasher boards and shattered his fourth and fifth cervical vertebrae.

Three hours later, Travis, Brenda, Lee and Tobi were told the worst. Travis would never be physically the same. He would never walk and most likely would never move his arms, hands, or fingers again. He would be a quadriplegic.

Thus began twenty-five years of peaks and valleys, hope and heartbreak, triumphs and defeats, victories and losses for Travis, our immediate family, extended family, and his and our close friends.

Because that night's game was being telecast, Travis' story became more than just another spinal cord injury (SCI) statistic. A video of his on-ice injury was broadcast live, and it quickly went viral. Within twenty-four hours, his accident had reached national, if not worldwide, exposure.

The impact of his story would eventually change the lives of thousands through his foundation, but at the time, it inspired thousands more to lend support to Travis and our family.

These "angels" carried not only Travis but all of us through those first difficult days, weeks, and months, and eventually to heights we never dreamed possible. The Travis Roy Foundation, created a year later, went on to raise more than $25 million for other SCI survivors and for research in search of a cure.

The injury to Travis devastated our world. Nothing prepares you for that kind of news. Now, what do you do?

You cry and you worry a lot, and you try to answer questions you never had to ask before. With the help of family, friends, caregivers, complete strangers, the video, and excellent insurance, we eventually began to learn, adjust, and move forward. What we didn't do was wallow in self-pity or dwell on the whys, how-comes, and what-ifs that we knew would only bring Travis and us down.

After surgery and 115 days at Boston University Medical Center, we determined that the best opportunity for Travis to move forward meant leaving the support of family and friends in Boston and moving to The Shepherd Center, an outstanding rehabilitation hospital in Atlanta, GA. Travis was medivacked to Atlanta, where he spent the next fifty-eight days trying to figure out how to live in a body incapable of movement or sensation.

After intense physical and occupational therapy, on April 13, 1996, Travis returned to our home in Yarmouth. When he left for Boston University the previous August, he had been in the best physical shape of his life. When he returned, for all intents and purposes, he had the body and needs of an infant. Mom and Dad were now caregivers.

While insurance provided for both aides and nursing care as needed, that wasn't always available. It became clear that family members would have to fill in.

In the evening and overnight, Travis preferred that we provide his care. The dinner meal was prepared by Brenda, and we quickly learned that she did a better job feeding Travis than Dad. There were fewer spills and less laundry. Putting Travis to bed was a shared responsibility. A mechanical device called a Hoyer lift, used to lift someone out of a power chair, made the transfer from chair to bed much easier. Dressing and undressing, bladder care, positioning, etc., eventually fell into a routine, and within an hour, Travis would be in bed for the night.

That didn't mean, as caregivers, we were through for the night, however. A baby monitor was used, and we took turns responding to his needs: scratch my nose, move my pillow, get me a drink, change the channel, or shut the TV off. There were very few nights that we were able to sleep through the night.

We made it through the first five months with a *lot* of trial and error. Accidents of every kind seemed to be a daily occurrence. It wasn't unusual to have to dress and undress Travis once or twice during the day. We got better at it, however, and learned, as Travis did, how often his leg bag needed to be emptied, when his pills needed to be administered, or that he needed repositioning because of a spasm. We learned Travis needed his alone time rather than having someone hover over him throughout the day. He needed space and a chance to be by himself. That was true for Mom and Dad as well. It took time to not only be comfortable with all this but also to articulate our individual needs to each other.

Fortunately, Travis was excellent at giving direction for his care. With the many aides and nurses that came into his life along with family members, this was a gift. "There is more than one way to do something" he would say, and we had to learn to defer to Travis. With so little that he could physically do for himself, it was important that we give him this control. This lesson took Mom and Dad a while to learn, and thankfully, Travis was infinitely patient.

"Mars vs. Venus" or the male vs. female perspective also played a role. Things that Mom worried about were often things Dad never even thought about, and vice versa. We had been married for twenty-six years and were just realizing how different we were. Fortunately for the two of us, but even more so for Travis, we adjusted and learned from each other. He became the beneficiary of both points of view. Between the three of us, we lived and learned every aspect of caring for a quadriplegic. We had to learn what was truly worthy of worry and what were routine idiosyncrasies of paralysis. We did our very best to ensure he had the best quality of life possible.

We started out as an immediate family of four: Mom, Dad, Tobi, and Travis. Effie (a Springer Spaniel) was also an important member. Two weeks after Travis returned to Yarmouth, his sister was married to Keith VanOrden. Neither has really been mentioned to this point, but both played integral roles in our getting through that first year and beyond.

Tobi was a second-year registered nurse, and Keith was newly employed in the field of finance. Fortunately for us, Tobi provided day-to-day awareness as to what was being done to and for Travis from a medical viewpoint. Almost immediately, Brenda and I asked Keith to be the spokesperson for the family, with all the media attention surrounding Travis' accident. Without the two of them providing for these two critical areas, Brenda and I would never have made it.

In the first 115 days at Boston Medical Center, after working an eight-hour shift as a neonatal nurse at Beth Israel Hospital, Tobi would arrive at Boston Medical to have dinner with us and spend time with her brother so we could have a break. After this, she would join other family members and friends who were spending hours each night responding to the hundreds of people who continued to send money and other forms of support for Travis and our family. Tobi was a pillar of strength that made such a difference for Travis, Brenda, and me.

Keith, meanwhile, had been thrown to the wolves. After his workday, he, too, would show up at the hospital and try to find time for dinner before responding via text, email, or phone calls to the various media outlets. With no training at all, Keith, like us, had to become a caregiver for us so that we could focus on Travis and survive each day. He was also our technology expert and spent one afternoon in the rain up on the roof of the hospital installing a satellite dish so Travis could get television coverage of a Boston University hockey game.

For the next twenty-five years, not only did Keith and Tobi continue to be caregivers in many ways, but their oldest daughter, Olivia, worked as Travis' aide for three summers. She did an excellent job learning a lot about caregiving, and the two of them formed a very special bond. Besides Olivia, close friends and cousins also became night caregivers during the summer months. This was obviously more fun for Travis than having strangers put him to bed at night. It gave him a sense of freedom, as well as allowing Mom and Dad to have weeknights off.

We would be remiss if we didn't give the Shepherd Center credit for what they did to support Travis and our family.

First, the Shepherd Center gave Travis the ability, knowledge, and tools to deal with his life as a quadriplegic. They showed and taught him that the only limitations as a quadriplegic were those he placed upon himself. He learned to paint using his mouth. He went into their pool with scuba equipment. He shot a gun with the use of a sip and puff. They arranged a field trip to the airport in Atlanta, where they showed us how to get him from his power chair

29

to an aisle chair to a seat on the plane. Travis learned that there was life as a quadriplegic.

Second, the Shepherd Center taught Brenda, Tobi, Travis's girlfriend Maija, and me how to do everything necessary for Travis' day-to-day care. We each completed a three-day course that had us physically doing his bowel and bladder care, feeding, dressing/undressing, using a Hoyer lift and slide board, and doing all the daily routines that he normally would perform for himself. Every question that a caregiver could think of was answered. Medical questions and concerns were discussed. Concerns particular to a quadriplegic were addressed. We all left these classes and the safety net of Shepherd feeling nervous but well-prepared to begin our new roles as caregivers.

From Travis' and our experience, here is another important tip for caregivers. We all have good days and bad, and some days just plain "suck" (excuse the language). If you are a caregiver who is having one of those days, don't bring it with you into the room. Put a smile on your face, and greet your loved one or patient with a positive attitude. Whoever you are a caregiver for, that person has probably had a worse day than you and doesn't need your troubles to add to their own. Be upbeat even when it's difficult. Bring joy rather than more discouragement or sadness into the room. A smile goes a long way to brighten everyone's day.

Once you learn to be a caregiver, those skills can be used in other situations as well. Nine years after Travis' accident, Brenda was diagnosed with breast cancer. Her best chance for survival was to have a double mastectomy. After surgery, many of those same caregiving skills that she and I had learned caring for Travis made it easier for me to help Brenda heal and move on with her life. Today (2022), she continues to enjoy good health and life.

There is an ending to our story. Travis, following surgery for bladder cancer, passed away from septic shock at the age of forty-five. His death on October 29, 2020, came twenty-five years, almost to the day after his accident. As parents, we are once again empty nesters. While he is finally free of his wheelchair and eternally at peace, we would give anything to be his caregivers again.

THE FOREVER PARENT

by *Maura Clow*

with *Mark J. Resnick*

I enjoyed a very normal pregnancy. I was 23 years old, physically fit, and healthy. *There's nothing I could have done differently.*

In the early morning hours of December 27, 1991, I delivered my firstborn child, Peter. Because he was a breached baby, it was C-Section delivery, but the doctor and nurses said there was no cause for concern. I would come to hear that phrase often in the coming years.

When the pediatrician returned the following day to check on us, I asked him about Peter's stiffness. His legs stood straight, and to swaddle him, you had to push his legs down. "There's not a lot of room in there while the baby waits to be born—no need to worry," he said.

Even though Peter was my first child, my husband Harry and I had lots of experience with babies, as both of us were the oldest of five kids in our families. Despite how tense Peter seemed, I was far more concerned about breastfeeding. My cousin gave birth to a daughter around the same time. We shared stories about our babies, and even though it was hard not to compare Peter's development to her daughter, she reminded me that girls develop differently than boys.

It wasn't until Peter was about six weeks old that I thought there might be something wrong with him. It was a photographer who clued me in. I remember him saying, "I do this all day long, and babies ought to be able to hold their heads up by this time."

Then, a few weeks later, after I went back to work, the owner of Peter's home-based daycare, a woman with 20 years of experience, started complaining about Peter. "He's not sleeping well, he has trouble holding his bottle, and he isn't crawling, like the others."

My pediatrician held firm. "You don't know yet; it's your first, and babies develop differently."

Harry's mom ran a daycare, so she came to see what the fuss was about. Her advice: "Don't let it go. Get another opinion." My aunt, a NIC unit nurse, did her own examination on Peter's first birthday. "You need to see a developmental pediatrician."

I'm not one to sit idle and hope for the best. I didn't know what, if anything, was wrong with Peter, but I wanted answers. This was no different than any other problem or challenge I faced in my life: if there was a problem, I needed to fix it. There was no internet or Google in 1992, but I was lucky to have a network of family nurses, and one of them introduced us to a developmental pediatrician in Albany, NY. Peter was 18 months old by the time we got an appointment with him.

The doctor conducted physical and developmental tests on Peter. He was thorough. "I don't know what this is, but I don't think you're going to be laughing about it later." In other words, this wasn't a *remember when little Johnny couldn't pronounce his R's* situation that families looked back upon with humor.

Something was wrong with Peter, but nobody knew what. He couldn't walk until he was 22 months old. He didn't talk. The following year, we took him to a geneticist. They did tons of testing on him. The doctor ruled out the genetic mutation called Fragile X. "He doesn't have Fragile X. This baby is fine."

We didn't stop there. We tested Peter for allergies. Nothing. Because he had lots of ear infections, they put tubes in his ears. His tonsils were removed. We tested his hearing for deafness. His eyes were checked to confirm his vision was fine. It was. An orthopedist did an entire body scan. We did a sleep-deprived EEG. All the while, we continued to see a developmental specialist.

Next, we took him to the neurologist to test for autism, even though it was not widely diagnosed in children this young at the time. "*Maybe,*" the doctor said. "But he interacts with you. He wants your attention—even engages with you. That's not typical with autism."

We drove from Albany, where we still lived, to Boston Children's Hospital to see more doctors. They said, "It's something, but we don't know what it is." Peter was a very social toddler, so he didn't fit the normal profile of autism. To add to my frustration, each time we visited Children's, it was a different set of doctors. By the time he was six, I had four different reports from four different specialists.

They ranged from *you ought to institutionalize him* to *he's totally fine*. One doctor told us: "He needs more floor time. He's fine; just play with him more." Seriously!

The first "break" we got was the discovery of a federally funded program—an early intervention school—normally reserved for 3-year-olds. I had to fight for it, but we got him into the school at 24 months. Instead of doing occupational and physical therapy at home, he was able to get it at the school. It was a huge help for us and Peter's development, but it still didn't provide any clear answer to the question: *what's wrong with my son?*

When he was four, we took Peter to the Bronx to see Dr. Isabelle Rapin. We waited two and a half hours after she completed her tests (with no toys, mind you) before she declared: He has Pervasive Development Disorder (PDD). *He has what?*

"What do we do about it?" I asked.

"There's nothing you can do—it's not going away."

"I have to try, though. There must be something we can do?"

"Nope, there's nothing."

Even my mom commented on how brutal Dr. Rapin's demeanor was. I was just glad to know what he had—that there was a name for it now. It took four years to get this far. Also, by this time, I had already had my daughter, Michaela, and still worked full-time. Harry travelled a lot for work, so it was an exhausting time for us both.

But there was no time to rest. Now that I knew what he had, sort of, I had to figure out what to do about it. I became a developmental specialist the old-fashioned way: using the Dewey decimal system in the library to locate medical journals. I read any and all articles, books, and journals on autism and PDD I could get my hands on.

We relied once again on our network of family nurses and friends to get us an appointment with Dr. Michael Powers in Connecticut. Nicknamed "The God of Autism," we were told he knew everything about autism. I prayed that he had some secret pill in his drawers to cure Peter.

"I can't cure Peter, but we can make his condition better."

Dr. Powers suggested we look into Applied Behavior Analysis (ABA) and the research conducted by Dr. Ivar Lovaas, a renowned psychologist and professor at UCLA. ABA teaches kids with autism how to communicate more efficiently through prompts, including flashcards, but it is somewhat controversial, too. Critics argued ABA would turn autistic kids into robots because the process prompted forced responses. See card A, automatically say card A.

But I had already tried everything up to this point and there was an ABA school 45 minutes away. Peter had to go through extensive ABA training before he could attend this specialized school. Four days a week, specialists came to the house to work with Peter to prepare him, but fortunately, the costs were covered by the School District.

Harry and I were also trained in ABA. It was important for the parents to be fully committed and prepared, so they could use and reinforce ABA at home. Unique to Peter's case, however, was that he couldn't talk until he was ten years old. As Dr. Powers later joked, "He has Peter Clow Syndrome!" When he was 18 months old I took multiple sign language classes and Peter and I would supplement his ABA training with signing. Harry learned to sign, too, and both of us read and signed Dr. Seuss books with Peter.

Learning the ABA system required Peter to study hundreds of laminated pictures. He would use whole strips of laminated cards to construct full sentences. At home, Peter would give me a laminated card to tell me what he wanted or needed.

Peter was 6 when we moved to Boston. Harry's career was thriving, but when job offers came, we had to turn most of them down. Unless a particular community had good special education programs, we couldn't even consider it. Basically, our current doctors advised against moving south of the Mason-Dixon line.

In 1998, we moved to Boston. We ultimately chose the town of Walpole because it was the only school district that worked with me prior to making our decision to move. I called dozens of school districts around Boston, and pretty much all of them said, "When you get here, we'll figure it out." NO, that was definitely not going to work. I needed to figure this out before we moved. I needed a plan. Walpole came through.

Peter had two siblings, Michaela and Harry III. Within a few years, Maeve and Richard were born. Walpole was a good choice for the entire family, not just Peter. Of course, each time I was expecting, I was a wreck. When I was expecting Richard, I had to spend four months in a hospital, on bed rest, prior to his birth. The support I received from the local community was extraordinary. Walpole friends, along with the parents and parishioners at Blessed Sacrament, helped Harry care for my entire family during my hospital stay.

Monday through Thursday, four girlfriends took the little ones from 2-6 p.m. Then people from the parish came to watch all the kids. These were complete strangers. The Blessed Sacrament first-grade class brought meals. And on and on it went, for four months. It was truly incredible.

We were lucky in more ways than one. Peter's doctors had warned us for years, "If he didn't speak by the time he was seven, he's not going to talk." Harry and I never believed that. We kept trying long after his seventh, eighth, and ninth birthdays. We got super lucky with his speech therapist. Without her, Peter probably never would have talked. Everybody who worked with Peter was great. His aids, teachers, and therapists pushed him—they set the bar higher and higher—and he exceeded those marks each time.

Peter did learn to talk. He was ten years old, but he did it. Between his therapists pushing him and his Dyna Box (a tablet similar to an iPad that translated symbols into speech), Peter found a way. It wasn't easy. Walpole's services were fantastic, but its summer program wasn't very robust. To prevent any regression, we had to find a program on our own outside of Walpole.

We found a camp in Westwood for children with autism, but the town refused to pay for it. We had to seek legal counsel to request that Walpole pay for camp, and ultimately, a mediator agreed that Walpole should pay for it. It was difficult fighting with the same people who were so accommodating all these years, but if you don't fight for services, you just don't get them.

Even before Peter began talking regularly, he could always say a couple of words...mom, dad, stop. But at camp, he started to talk more. His gross motor skills got so much better that it allowed his fine motor skills to develop. And he kept talking and going to speech therapy. By the time he turned eleven, he no longer needed his speech therapy box.

On a family trip to Disneyworld, I remember shouting, "Peter, would you shut up! Be quiet for a few minutes." Then, the whole family would give it right back to me. "Mom, remember when you used to pray for him to talk!"

Peter's teen years were difficult. Autistic or not, boys have hormones. There was a lot of inappropriate talk and missed social cues for Peter. Crowds were especially hard to maneuver, as he would often create a scene. It was hard on the whole family. The impact on his siblings was great, but Harry and I were determined not to have their lives diminished because of a special needs sibling. As my dad so accurately reminded me, "He's your kid, not your cause." And he was right. We never wanted our family defined by Peter's disability and did our best to follow through on that goal.

Yet, there's no escaping the fact that a person with autism requires continuous management and care. Peter aged out of his summer camp at age 13, so we had to find an alternative camp solution. Dr. Powers suggested a sleepaway camp. He said Peter needed to learn how to be away from me and me from him. His long-term growth depended on his development of this skill. Peter's transition to a group home would take place years from now, but the reality is it takes years to prepare for it.

Unfortunately, we had to fight with the school district again to get them to pay for a sleepaway camp. Another sad reality with special education is that the only way to prove you're right is to sacrifice your child and let them fail. If Peter was unable to go to summer camp, the chances of him regressing were high. But I was not going to sacrifice Peter and let him fail just to prove to Walpole that I was right. We fought hard once again, to the tune of $50,000 in legal fees.

It's possible the school district didn't want to pay for it because, in part, they thought we were trying to get him into a group home early. And if that happened, they would be on the hook for that expense until he turned 22. This would not be a good precedent to set. But that wasn't the case at all. His prior camp experiences were the very opposite of regression—he thrived each and every year—whether it was his speech, social interactions, or dependency skills.

It was another battle. Exhausting and expensive, but worth every penny.

I was so nervous for Peter prior to his departure that first summer, but he hopped out of the car and said, "So long, suckers!" and got on the bus. I cried, but the tears were happy ones. It was the best thing we ever did for Peter. No, it was the best thing I ever did for myself. I had to learn to live without him. I didn't realize just how much space in my brain was allocated to taking care of Peter. My first thought each morning was always how to manage around him, but for seven weeks, that planning wasn't required. Peter's sleepaway camps allowed us to do things as a family that we couldn't do with Peter. There was no guilt either, as Peter was having the time of his life at these camps. As a family, we couldn't be equal in terms of experiences and attention, but we could be—and were—equitable in this regard.

Dr. Powers' other critical piece of advice was to get Peter into residential care ASAP. "Do not delay it." Walpole's Turning 22 program ended at age 22, at which point the school district services ended, and it was time for adults with autism to enter a group home. Unfortunately, families who don't heed this advice find it increasingly difficult to find a placement in one of these homes. There simply aren't enough of them, but more importantly, all the skills regarding self-dependency get lost the longer a family delays this decision.

I began investigating houses when Peter was eighteen. I met with the Commonwealth to determine what level of care he needed, and because I started the process so early, Peter was at the top of the list when he turned 22.

Because we asked for it. Because we fought for it. They aren't going to hand it to you; you have to fight for it.

So yes, having a child with autism means you're a parent forever. Even when they enter a group home, you need to stay on top of things, whether it's the home's standard of cleanliness, staff transitions, or ensuring he has the necessary items we want him to have. Peter's pretty good at doing things for himself, but if he doesn't, you need to make sure he gets them done. We can't control how his brain works, but we can control how he looks, whether that means how often he is shaving and showering or how clean his clothes are. Equally as important, Peter's not going to complain about anything inside the home, so again, that falls on the parents or guardians to be on top of things.

Caring for Peter has taught me so much about myself. I had to learn to give up control over the things I couldn't control, which is one of the hardest things I've had to do in my life. I'm a pretty in-control person—I like things the way I like things. Peter also needed consistency, something that is important for all autistic kids and adults. You can't always be there for them to provide that consistency, though. I had to pretend I was Scarlet O'Hara—every time I got sad, I said I couldn't think about it.

Life doesn't treat you any differently just because you have a child with special needs. When we feared Harry might lose his job, I said God wouldn't do that to me. I relied on the phrase, "God doesn't give you more than you can handle..." Right, well, yes—sometimes he does. When Harry did lose his job, we were entering the most expensive four years of our lives. Peter was 22, Michaela was in college, Harry was in a private high school, and my youngest two were in a private elementary school.

Somehow, we did handle it.

Having a child with autism is like winning a lottery, even though you never purchased a ticket. This was a lottery you didn't want to win—nobody hopes to have a special needs child. But you learn to adapt.

Years ago, I read a *Dear Abby* article about a family who was planning this amazing trip to Italy, with all the excursions you would dream of taking. Only their plane landed in Holland instead, so they did things differently. It was slower in Holland but just as beautiful. Different but just as amazing. She likened it to having a special needs child. Plans change, but like a Marine, you need to improvise, adapt, and overcome. You can't control everything, no matter how hard you try.

You rely on family, friends, your own children, and sometimes strangers—like I had to do when bed-ridden during Richard's pregnancy. I was never very good at asking for help, but caring for Peter made me better at accepting help, and I'm glad I did. We've been given a lot of grace and help from the community of Walpole. Our kids have seen that generosity and will hopefully return that grace in return.

Harry and I did our best to provide equitable opportunities for growth and happiness for all five of our children. We never wanted them to feel overshadowed by Peter's special needs and believe we succeeded in that goal. My kids are happy. I know Peter is. He loves living in a group home. He comes home most weekends but always looks forward to returning.

I'm grateful to my dad, who reminded me that Peter was my son—not my cause, and my mother for teaching me not to take no for an answer. I'm grateful to my children, who loved and supported Peter at every turn—but never let his needs and desires define who they were or what they were capable of becoming. I am grateful for our family and friends who accommodated and accepted Peter, and kept inviting The Clow Clan into their lives and homes. And I'm grateful to my husband Harry—for always letting me *be me*, even when there were many times, I'm sure, he wished I was someone else!

Come to think of it...*there's nothing I would have done differently.*

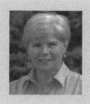 Maura Clow lives in Walpole, MA with her charming husband, Harry. Her greatest joy is being a mother to Peter, Michaela, Harry III, Maeve & Richard.

LIVING WITH DEMENTIA: A JOURNEY

by Jane Dwinell

"I think this is going to be harder for you than for me." These were the first words out of Sky's mouth once we reached the sanctuary of our car.

My husband, Sky Yardley, had just been diagnosed with "probable early-stage Alzheimer's." He was sixty-six and in otherwise perfect health.

We held hands on the short drive home, not speaking, both of us silently crying. Even though I knew this diagnosis was coming, it was still a shock. I was sad and stunned, but I was also relieved to finally have an answer. I had watched Sky's short-term memory and spatial skills disappear over the previous year, and as an RN who had worked in a memory care facility, I was sure it was dementia. And so it was.

Fortunately, Sky embraced his diagnosis and began to read everything he could get his hands on about dementia. He wanted to find "his people" and began attending the local Memory Cafe. He started writing about life with dementia—both as a way to make sense of what was happening to him, but also to share his reality on our blog, Alzheimer's Canyon. He went about town in the "brain hat" that I had knitted for him. He used it as a conversation starter when people said, "Hey! I like your hat!" Sometimes, people wanted to talk about their experience with a loved one with dementia, but mostly people walked away.

Some family and friends drifted away. A few dear ones hung in with us, visiting, hiking and biking with Sky, playing games, going out for lunch with me, and keeping in touch via email and phone calls. Our world began to shrink as Sky began to be anxious about just about everything— a 180-degree turn from the laid-back, calm man I had known for so long.

At first, there was little for me to "do" other than to keep my eye on Sky, answer his questions, smooth the way when he was scared, and remind him of anything special we were doing that day. Our life went on as it had—days spent walking, boating, biking and gardening, meals together, reading, crossword puzzles, and evenings spent watching movies or playing Bridge or board games with our son and his partner.

Fortunately for us, Sky and I had retired early, in our mid-fifties, so we could travel and do volunteer work. Clearly, those days were over, but we were grateful that we had had so many adventures, knowing that most people retire in their mid-sixties—just when Sky was diagnosed. He had done everything he wanted to do—there was no "bucket list" to complete. Now, he just wanted to do what he could to erase the stigma of a dementia diagnosis.

So we began public speaking, leading workshops and worship services, talking to college students, and being on public panels about dementia. All of this brought Sky such joy—he was connecting with "his people" as we traveled around the country.

Then the hallucinations began.

Day in and day out, Sky communed with the natural world—with the tree spirits, the young maidens dancing in the fields, the sprites that lived in our backyard, and the dolphins that swam in our northern lake. He was so frustrated that the rest of us couldn't see these creatures. Sometimes, the hallucinations turned dark when he feared someone in the family was hurt or dead, or that the police were outside, or that the water main had broken and the house was being flooded. The hallucinations came and went, but they were most frequent at night.

That meant I was getting very little sleep.

I was doing fine with helping Sky dress, bathe, and find the bathroom in the middle of the night. It was getting harder to find things for him to do during the day as his skills began to drop away. Bridge and board games were out, as were reading and bike riding. He listened to audio books, watched nature documentaries, and took long walks—until he got lost and couldn't find his way home. His world—and mine—got smaller and smaller.

Miraculously, he was still writing. But lack of sleep began to wear on me. Sky would fall right back to sleep after his various bathroom trips in the night, but I usually didn't. Sometimes, he would wake me up to tell me about his latest hallucination (good or bad), and once again, he would fall back to sleep, and I wouldn't. Our son and I began to trade off nights, but that made Sky worse as he was sure I was dead. Our son finally said, "I didn't realize that taking care of Sky would mean we wouldn't be able to sleep."

Our local memory care facility offered a respite program—someone could stay for two weeks to two months to give the family a break. Sky and I visited for a day. He attended activities while I talked with the staff and observed their interactions with the residents. Sky agreed to go for a time of respite so that I could sleep. I dropped him off on March 10, 2020, and two weeks later, we went into lockdown because of COVID-19.

My caregiving days were over, but I didn't realize it at the time. No one knew what was going to happen with the pandemic. But it became clear before too long that Sky was going to stay at the facility for the indefinite future. The staff—despite trying different medications—had not found the answer to Sky's hallucinations and nighttime shenanigans. I was just as happy to let them deal with his wandering, incontinence, and hallucinations. But I missed him terribly.

Nearly a year after I dropped Sky off at the facility, it was clear that he was dying. Pandemic or no pandemic, I was allowed to be at his side as he transitioned from this world to the next. The staff cared for me as they cared for him, bringing me a cot and meals, as well as telling me stories of Sky's various hallucinatory adventures. He was in and out of consciousness for three days but always knew me when he was awake. He was still singing, and the last time he was awake, he said, "The end is near."

It was a gift to be able to partner with Sky as he embraced his diagnosis, handled it with as much grace as he could, and trusted me deeply. But he was right. It was harder for me than for him. It was incredibly painful to lose the man I had loved for thirty-six years, watch his gifts and skills fade away, watch anxiety take over from calm, and watch him become a diminished Sky.

But his greatest fear did not come true—he was still him; he did not lose his essential self. And there was a twinkle in his eye when he said his last words to me: "You are so beautiful."

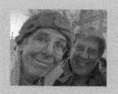 Jane Dwinell is the author of four books, most recently *Alzheimer's Canyon: One Couple's Reflections on Living with Dementia* (Rootstock Publishing, 2022) co-authored with her late husband, Sky Yardley. In addition to being an author, she is a retired RN and Unitarian Universalist minister. She lives in northern Vermont with her two cats and her garden. She is available for public speaking and workshops. Contact her through janedwinell.com.

IT'S ON ME

by Marisa Boidi

I t's 3:00 a.m., and I'm awake—because I'm a caregiver. Sleep has become a thing of the past, just like so many other things.

Have you ever woken up one day and had your life change forever? You had all these plans: a successful career, a beautiful home, two beautiful children, a loving husband, no debt, and then, one moment changes everything. For me, that was what we call "D" day. The day my two-and-a-half-month-old daughter was diagnosed with a rare disease called Spinal Muscular Atrophy Type 1 (SMA). It's known as the number one genetic killer of infants. At that moment, it was like a piece of me died; it felt like my heart was ripped out of my chest and stomped on over and over again.

How could this be? No child should have to suffer this fate.

SMA is a disease in which the body is missing the gene that produces SMN protein, and that protein is what keeps the motor neurons alive. Over time, my daughter's motor neurons would die, and her muscles would atrophy. People with the disease lose the ability to walk, swallow, and eventually breathe. As the doctors explained this, it hit me—if all of her muscles would atrophy, would she be able to smile or talk—what would happen to her— would she suffer? As we were told, historically, yes. But a new drug was just approved by the FDA that had great promise to stop the progression of the disease.

It was at that very moment I turned my pain into hope. Are there times I want to drown in self-pity? Of course. I'm only human. But do I? Absolutely not. I've always feared that if I sat too long in sadness, I might not recover. Maybe spending too much time with what makes me sad would make us miss what would make us happy. I knew I needed to be strong for my daughter. It was time to fight. So I dusted myself off and haven't looked back.

Did I know at that moment how hard this life was going to be? Nope, I had no clue. Being a caregiver is the hardest yet most important job you will ever have. You couldn't possibly understand the emotional and physical impact on you until you are actually a caregiver.

My life is hard. I'm a mother of two young kids, one of whom is considered medically fragile and disabled. I work full-time. I do all the things a wife and mother does, and I also play the role of nurse, physical therapist, and advocate. To say I'm exhausted is an understatement, but just like every new mom, your body adjusts. You find your way through this new life, and as you navigate, you learn to cope, too.

Because of my daughter's disease, I've been gifted with the ability to see life differently now. I've witnessed a true fight, passion, and love—unconditional and never-ending love. I've seen family, friends, and community come together to fight for a little girl most have never met. We have raised more than $200,000 for SMA research in the last five years. That is nothing short of amazing.

Strangers have offered to give her money for a Make-A-Wish trip because they said just meeting her while waiting for a vaccine was so impactful to them. They wanted this little girl to have the best time of her life. She has not only opened my eyes to what's important but the eyes of people she's never met. With her positivity, drive, and stubbornness, she shows the world every day she won't be told what she can't do, and her spirit inspires.

It's hard to put into words what it feels like when you finally accept your child's diagnosis. You still never give up hope that they will live longer and have a happy life, but you come to terms with the diagnosis.

She keeps me going each day. Every birthday and every milestone is a moment I cherish. Every day is a new lesson on life for me.

My life now is about giving her the best quality of life possible. Letting her experience things other children do. She will need to do it differently, but she will do it and she will smile like she always does. There is no time for self-pity or rest. The clock isn't on our side; there is lots to do and lots of joyous and memorable moments to be had. She needs me, and I need her. Each day she reminds me, *Mama, you are my best friend.* And each day, it melts my heart. Being a caregiver is so tiring at times, but watching my daughter smile and laugh makes it all worth it. They said she won't have a life, and I gave her one.

As a caregiver, you have so much more responsibility and so many more worries. But if you take the time to see past that, you will see that you were blessed—not with the perfect life—but with seeing the world in a way most won't or can't. I've met so many amazing and selfless people through this journey. I've truly seen the best of the human spirit, and there are no words to describe it. It's beautiful.

I've learned that people can't truly understand the intensity of being a caregiver. They would never understand your fears. For me, being my daughter's caregiver means it's on me to keep her alive. I'm not a nurse, doctor, or an EMT. I'm a project manager. It's not a role I would have expected to play, but here I am. Instead of getting upset or mad each time I feel like someone doesn't understand or says something hurtful, I've tried to turn it into a teaching moment. I'm human, and I still get offended or get sad, but like I said before, I don't stay there. There is no time in this journey to sit with bad feelings. Sure, take a moment and feel it at times. But then dust yourself off quickly. Get back up—someone is depending on you.

When you're feeling your worst, it's time for a break. Find someone you can trust to step in for a couple hours, and then get some shopping therapy, do your nails, golf, or just sleep. It's deserved and required. You need to be mentally and physically fit for this job. I find that writing can be helpful when I feel overwhelmed. Even if I don't share the words, it has helped clear my head. I also have joined many social media groups for other caregivers and have spent time helping nonprofits that have helped me. At times, it might feel like taking a moment for yourself is selfish, but it's not.

If you're the mother of a child with special needs, you may already be familiar with Emma Bombeck's poem, *The Special Mother.* Each time I feel bad about doing something for myself, or I feel like I'm failing, I read it to remind myself I was chosen for all these reasons—and I need to be kinder to myself. I'm doing the best I can.

Marisa Boidi is a seasoned Client Service, IT, & Project Management professional with an impressive track record spanning over 20 years. Her dedication doesn't stop there – Marisa is also a devoted mother, raising two children with her husband in Eastern Massachusetts. Marisa's life took a transformative turn when her youngest daughter was diagnosed with Spinal Muscular Atrophy (SMA), a rare disease that led her to become a passionate advocate for SMA awareness and research. While juggling the demands of her career with the role of primary caregiver, Marisa also works tirelessly to raise awareness and funds for SMA.

WITHOUT LOVE, CAREGIVING IS JUST A CHORE

by Riva Scher

with Mark J. Resnick

My daughter, Debra, was born with juvenile rheumatoid arthritis, commonly known as JRA. Although she wasn't formally diagnosed until her second birthday, there was obviously something very wrong with her by the time she began walking. Debra walked on her toes, as if walking flat on her feet was not possible. Also, she was normally a sweet and quiet child, but the mere touch of her feet would cause her to scream in pain.

The pediatrician dismissed my concerns, but thankfully, my husband's colleague referred us to an allergist. He knew right away that she had JRA, which is a disease of the joints and cartilage, and it carries with it a crippling effect. In children, it can impact one joint or many joints. In her case, it was every joint. Debra's joints became so crippled that there were many times she couldn't walk or move her hands. When her joints crippled that badly, the doctors would straighten them out with surgery.

The pediatric oncologist who gave us the JRA diagnosis initially thought Debra had cancer. Her life was so tortuous that I'm not so sure it wouldn't have been better if she had cancer. With cancer, at least there was the possibility of remission or an outright cure. With her JRA, she lived the most painful life. Thirty-five major surgeries in twenty-six years. More than one per year.

By the time she was sixteen, she already had two surgeries on her jaw. The first one required the surgeon to reconstruct the jaw from her pelvic bone. The second surgery was to implant a new chin. Following the surgeries, Debra's jaw was wired shut, and she was fed through a nasogastric tube for six months each time.

It was always a challenge helping Debra manage her pain. She had a daily regimen of twenty-five baby aspirin. Bayer, the aspirin manufacturer, shipped us the drugs for free. There wasn't much else we could do for the pain. She tried some experimental drugs, but those didn't work. One of them involved the injection of gold—actual gold. That didn't work. Nothing worked.

To complicate her condition, Debra was diagnosed with Marfan syndrome at age twelve. Marfan syndrome is a disease of the collagen in the body. It affects the fibers—the connective tissues—which support the organs in your body, including the heart. It also affects the eyes, blood vessels, skin, lungs, and skeleton. Generally, people don't live past thirty. Although Debra is part of that statistic, it wasn't the syndrome that ultimately caused her death.

Debra could do very little by herself. First thing in the morning, just to get her to move, I gave her a warm bath. But really, she spent half of her life in the hospital or rehab center, doing pool therapy, occupational therapy, or physical therapy. The hospital was in Hollywood, CA, about an hour away from our home. There were times she would have to spend three, four, or five months in the hospital, especially before surgery. I spent most of my days at the hospital, doing things only moms can do.

Debra's older sister had a difficult time dealing with the attention given to her sick sibling. The limelight as the only child was snatched away from her. Additionally, she had to deal with the guilt of being healthy. When you're sharing a bedroom with someone who cries all night, who's in pain all the time, it's very hard.

My son, who was three years younger than Debra, handled it differently. He had ways to compensate for the attention given to Debra, whether it was his circle of friends or the sports he played.

Caregiving is the hardest job in the world, especially when there's little or no cure for what ails your loved one. At one point, Debra herself didn't have the will to live. We found a letter addressed to us, basically saying she didn't want to hurt us but that she didn't think she could live like this anymore. She was in and out of the hospital, missing school, having surgery after surgery.

Then, one day, while Debra was in Children's Hospital recovering from one of her many surgeries, a personal and confidential letter addressed to Debra arrived. Because it was addressed to her, we let her open it. The letter stated that the Children's Hospital would garnish her father's wages if we didn't pay a $6,000 bill that the insurance company had denied.

She read it, went to the bathroom, and tried to cut her wrists.

The very next day, Children's Hospital transferred her to a mental facility, the first of many institutions she endured over the next four years because she was suicidal. She spent time in six facilities and had one-on-one coverage outside her door at each one. Finally, when she was twenty, a doctor recognized that she was on fourteen different drugs. He sent her to a hospital in Arizona and adjusted her medication, removing all her psychotropic drugs. Thirty days later, she was released and back home, a completely different person. It was the first time in four years we recognized her as the Debra we knew.

No amount of compensation could justify the harm done by the insurance company, but needless to say, a judge in California issued the largest bad-faith settlement award to that point. Debra never had a normal life after her experience in the mental hospital, but she gave it her all to live an independent life from then on. With the settlement money, we bought her a condo and cared for her at her house. For a small stretch of time, she was even able to drive and get a job. Debra worked for a year until her pain became too severe, but she was so proud of herself for pushing forward.

Watching your daughter suffer—watching anybody you love suffer—is the absolute worst. My husband and I knew we could lose Debra at any time. Marfan syndrome and JRA are cruel diseases. But neither one was responsible for her ultimate demise at the young age of twenty-six.

Five days before her death, Debra was in the hospital for yet another surgery, this time on her knee. She told me they were going to kill her in the hospital, as she saw them make many mistakes. Her comments scared me, but she was pretty sure of it.

"Mom, you have to promise me you'll finish our book," she said.

We started writing a resource guide for parents of disabled children a while back. It was a cautionary tale for parents on what to expect and how to make the best of their situation. Of course, I made that promise, but only if she would stop worrying about dying in the hospital.

The knee surgery went well, but the morphine and valium that were administered post-surgery depressed her breathing. Debra was hooked up to an apnea monitor to alert the nursing staff when she stopped breathing. On the last evening of her life, we noticed the apnea monitor was outside her door and requested that they put it back. They told us they would have to get an order from the doctor to do that. We trusted they would get it done and left for the evening. They never did, and our Debra died overnight at 3:00 a.m.

The official cause was labeled an "accidental death," but it was really an overdose of morphine and valium that killed her. Without the monitor present, nobody realized that she had stopped breathing, and she became brain-dead.

When people think of caregiving, they don't always think of advocacy, which is every bit as important as administering medication, bathing, feeding, and clothing a loved one. I pleaded with the nursing staff to put the apnea monitor back and trusted that they would comply. I never should have trusted them; I never should have left that evening without seeing that it had been done.

I can't blame myself for not staying. After twenty-six years of intense hospitalizations, surgeries, pain, and suffering, my husband and I were paralyzed by exhaustion. Had this been her first surgery or fifth, there's no question we would have stayed, but long-term caregiving is an exhausting process, and as such, our minds weren't always able to track and capture every detail or request in her daily care.

In chapter two of my book, *Finally Dancing: A Bittersweet Odyssey*, I wrote about the night Debra died.

At 3:30 a.m., the shrill ringing of the phone cut through our sleep like a white-hot knife. We knew it had to be the hospital—it couldn't be good news. The voice at the other end said, "Come right now!" I hung up, not taking the time to ask any questions.

We dressed and drove in a blur, arriving at the hospital shortly after 4:00 a.m. We rushed to her fifth-floor room to find it empty, the bed stripped of its sheets and the apnea monitor still where it had been when we left the night before—outside the door.

Panicked and unsure what to do next, Sandy and I breathlessly approached the nurse's station, where we were directed upstairs to the intensive care unit.

Our greatest fears had been realized. The unthinkable had happened. Debby had stopped breathing. She lay still, a respirator and feeding tubes keeping her alive. She was not in a coma; she had been pronounced brain-dead.

I stood at her bedside, stroking Debby's cool brow. Against her colorless skin, the scattering of freckles on her face seemed more prominent. One of the nurses had braided her hair into pigtails. I knew I might never have another opportunity to be alone with my daughter. With all my senses, I drank in her essence, committing every inch of her slender, fragile body to memory.

I focused on her tattoos. Debby had two tattoos, one of a small yellow rose on her right ankle and the other of a tiny bluebird just above her breastbone. She had gotten them, against her father's wishes, because, as she said, "I have so many scars on my body; I just want something beautiful." She looked so young—she was so young. At twenty-six, Debby was much too young to die.

I could not let her go. The doctors made it perfectly clear to us that the brain activity had ceased, but it took me most of the day to process that fact. I understood intellectually, but as her mother, I held on as tightly as I could. I believed, no, I felt certain that if I waited long enough, she would wake up. Sitting by her bedside, holding her hand, I became even more certain that she was coming back to us when an involuntary muscle reflex caused her hand to move within mine.

Finally, after fifteen long, miserable hours, assured by both the neurologist who had been called in and Sandy, who understood the mechanics of brain death, I reluctantly gave in and acknowledged that there was not even a shred of hope. Without activity in the brain stem, Debby could not come back from the vegetative state she was in. Once I had accepted that fact, I knew Debra would not want to live like that. She so loved her independence . . . I had to let her go.

With the exception of those four years of mental anguish, and despite her terrible pain and afflictions, Debra had the most beautiful, positive, and mellow mindset. She handled everything the diseases threw at her, one surgery at a time. She was an amazing person.

Finishing the book was therapeutic only in the sense that I fulfilled my promise to Debra. It was a painful process but worth it because of the personal growth I got out of it and the people I met along the way. Writing expanded my horizons in ways I never imagined.

Caring for Debra was a blessing. She was a gift. I would give anything to go back and be with her again. And my husband—he was the most loving, patient, and amazing man. He was responsible for Debra's physical therapy at night. After working his two or three jobs, he came home, ate dinner, and worked with Debra.

Caregiving is a labor of love. It is not a punishment, job, or chore. No matter the circumstance or situation you're dealing with, without love, it's not caregiving—it's a chore.

It was never a chore for me.

 Riva Scher is a mother, grandmother, and now great-grandmother. Her book, *Finally Dancing: A Bittersweet Odyssey*, was published in 2021 to help families navigate long-term chronic illnesses and is available on Amazon. She has advocated for disabled students in public education as a member of the Los Angeles Unified School District's special education commission and the parent advisory committee for the superintendent of special education. Her roadshow on mainstreaming won a State of California award for volunteerism.

THE SHIT SHOW

by Candy Kavanagh

with Mark J. Resnick

I have always been a *shit happens* kind of person—meaning I don't dwell on the negative or rattle easily when faced with obstacles. I believe in meditation, spiritual balance, love, and remaining optimistic when everything you're faced with seems impossible. These are my beliefs, which have helped me overcome anything thrown at me during the fifty-one years I've been on this planet. But believe me when I say this: my take on the oft-used *shit happens* expression changed dramatically in 2016, when, nine months into a relationship with Tim Kavanagh, we learned he had colorectal cancer.

Having turned fifty in May, Tim scheduled a routine colonoscopy. Only it was anything but routine. In the middle of the procedure, Tim came out of his anesthesia-induced state and saw them removing something. In recovery, still loopy from the procedure, he saw how the nurse looked at him, and he knew there was a problem.

The nurse called me and asked if I could come to the recovery room when I arrived. That's when Tim told me he had cancer. I thought he was still under the effects of anesthesia and was thinking our worst nightmare was true, but it couldn't possibly be. "The doctor is coming back to talk to us," he said. I saw the look on his face—the look of fear on his face—and knew he was completely lucid. The shit show had just begun, and I had no idea what I was getting myself into.

Tim and I were both volunteering at an event when we met. He was a local entertainer with his own show on the CBS affiliate station and well known in the area. I knew who he was, but not the other way around. We were given walkie-talkies at the event, and Tim was told that I, Candy, had the other one. When the large crowd began to get antsy and wanted to know when they could be seated, I stood on a chair and asked how many knew who Tim Kavanagh was. To preface this next bit, Tim is 6'2", bald, and broad-shouldered. He also has the best smile and twinkling eyes you've ever laid eyes on, but that doesn't really apply to the story—it's just yet another thing to love about Tim. With the crowd cheering their admiration for Tim, I let them know he was on the other talkie. I clicked the button on the side and said, "Baldie Locks, I've got a code red in the front." He replied, "That's a big 10–4 Candy Cane." It was the start of a beautiful friendship, which blossomed into a romantic relationship over time.

Tim's medical team told us that he had stage 1 or 2 cancer, so he underwent chemotherapy and radiation at our local hospital and was a candidate for the Opera trial. The trial was successful for many, but not for Tim. The chemo shrank the tumor enough for surgery. After much deliberation, we decided to travel out of state to a well-known hospital so that an experienced doctor could perform the surgery that would remove 90% of his rectum and then do a temporary ileostomy.

Unfortunately, this was a teaching hospital, and even though I specifically requested the doctor perform the surgery and not a student, it was obvious my request was not granted. The ostomy was supposed to look like a rose but instead looked like a football. The difference is major when it comes to ostomies, and the complications were intense.

After the surgery, which took place right before the July Fourth holiday, the medical team wanted to discharge Tim. He was in no shape to be discharged. That much was obvious, but because of the holiday, they insisted he would be better off at home (which, in our case, was his brother's place since we were out of state). It wasn't really a choice, so I asked the nurse to load me up with supplies or I would pilfer from the supply closet for our long weekend. I left with six large bags and little idea how we would manage his care.

Thankfully, Tim's mother, Judy, a retired nurse, was on deck to help. Because of Tim's deformed ostomy, nothing could have prepared or helped either of us care for Tim. After the ileostomy, the bags attached to him were supposed to last three to four days per bag, but instead, I had to change them every twenty minutes. I will spare you the details, but it was at this time I leaned into my emotions and was at the "wailing wall" of despair.

On Tuesday, when we went for our checkup, my hair was unwashed, and I was frantic and frazzled after a horrifying four days. They examined Tim and were ready to send him home again. I told them point-blank, *Look at me. I can't take care of him. He has to be admitted.* I then gave them a list and told them they needed to check every single box before they released him. The list included things like walking three times around the hall without assistance and the ability to dress himself. I'm usually a straightforward person, but I found myself cursing at them. I was frustrated and threatened to speak with the administration if they wouldn't accept my checklist.

As a caregiver, you have to be ready to go there—to say whatever you have to say, in whatever manner you need to say it, to get anybody to listen to you. It blew my mind that I had to be this tough bitch before they said, "I guess she really means it." Tim was readmitted and was in the hospital for another four days, and yet, it was still a disastrous experience when we got home. Tim had third-degree burns from the bags not being attached properly, and according to our home health nurse, it was one of the top three worst ostomies she had ever seen in her twenty-eight years of nursing.

Up until this time, I had modified our diet and was mothering Tim more than being his sweetheart. I researched alternative methods, and we practiced our mantra of positive energy and instilled lots of love and humor to heal both of us, physically and mentally. I thought caregiving was mostly about emotional support, and it is, but it's so much more. The exhaustion, fear, uncertainty, and confusion are just a small part of it. *Sometimes, those are the easy parts.*

The end result of Tim's first surgery: the cancer seeded on the surgical opening, which led to the cancer spreading to his abdomen. I could write a whole book on the next three years—the pain, disappointment, fear, acceptance, grief, and our "together we can handle anything that comes our way" attitude—just to be pulled back down and begin the cycle all over again.

Moving into the fourth year of our cancer journey, 2020, Tim and I still walked five miles a day, ate well, meditated, laughed, loved, and enjoyed life. We did those things in spite of visiting the ER every month to fix his ongoing problems from the initial surgery.

On a high note, in July, under the willow trees in our backyard, he asked me to be his wife. Without hesitation I said, yes. Our lives were full of optimism and joy. We spent time with family and friends, snuggled with our dog, Adora, tackled household improvements, ran mundane errands, and dealt with a multitude of side effects in which the cancer had dealt.

This continued until a routine walk went awry. About a half mile from home, Tim said he had to lay on the grass and couldn't go any further. For him to say and act that way, I knew something was very wrong. He had pushed through *everything* and never complained.

I ran home, drove back to him, got him in the car, and sped off to the hospital. They admitted him for more scans and labs and sent me home. The next morning, I called Tim at 7:00 a.m., and he sounded tired but good. Feeling a bit relieved, I said I would bring my work to the hospital and see him later that morning. When I walked in at 8:30 a.m., he was clinging to the bed rail and begging me to help him. He was white, eyes large with terror and pain. His bowel had perforated; he was septic and needed emergency surgery.

Although Tim successfully championed surgery again and was discharged several days afterward, he wasn't himself. He napped a lot, and his complexion looked gray. His spirits were low—I was very concerned. October 10 was our wedding day, and I wondered if he would be able to stand and say his vows in front of our fifty closest friends and family. The COVID-19 pandemic was already a factor in threatening our wedding day, but his health was a much more distressing issue for me at the time.

I'm happy to say we were able to have our beautiful wedding day. The sun shone brightly, our friends and family gathered in our masks, and we exchanged vows and declared our love. The wind blew with great, cleansing energy, and we celebrated the breaking of glass as champagne flutes flew to the ground. Tim needed to leave the reception early, but we had our special day.

The memories from our wedding day gave us something to hold onto, and I can't tell you how many times we've recounted them in order to get through what was to come next.

A week later, the hospital where Tim had surgery in September experienced a cyberattack. All patient records were gone. Records of his treatment were gone. Thankfully, Tim had a team at the world-renowned Memorial Sloan Kettering Cancer Center in New York City. We trusted them implicitly and immediately passed all of Tim's care to them.

The doctors at Sloan diagnosed the issue of Tim's recent discomfort, which was an infection from the bowel perforation that had hardened. Tim's bladder had thankfully taken on the Herculean role of shielding the infection from traveling throughout his body, but as a result, his bladder and kidneys were damaged, and his ureters were crushed.

A December surgery was planned to remove the cancer in the abdomen and clean out the infection. We would be in NYC over Christmas. With dark humor we thought, because of COVID-19, what a perfect year for this to happen, as we wouldn't be able to be with our families anyway.

The surgery was expected to take fifteen hours, and recovery was projected to take eight weeks. As it turned out, we were in NYC until the beginning of March, almost double the time expected. The reason for the extended time frame was that Tim needed two surgeries a week to deep clean the area of infection and home health care every other day to irrigate and cleanse the wound. Tim had a state-of-the-art wound vac that pumped out the infection and expedited healing time. Only certified, highly trained, and skilled nurses were allowed to change and reattach the wound vac.

Now remember, it was COVID-19 in NYC, where the virus was raging. My mind filled with doubt and fear, wondering what we would do if the virus prevented Tim's trained nurses from coming. Just in case, I videotaped the nursing team while they cleaned his wounds, even though they firmly told me

I was not to try and change the wound vac myself. I nodded, saying it was the last thing I wanted to do—unless there was no other choice.

You guessed it. We ran out of choices when the home health nurse was unable to make it, and my husband was in desperate need of attention. We looked at each other, tears spilling down our faces, and I asked him, "Can you trust me?" But not before I turned my back, stared at the wall, and said to myself and my higher power, *If this is what you really want me to do, give me the strength to do this.*

Sometimes, you don't have a choice, and sometimes, this is when caregiving is *not knowing what you're doing but doing it anyway.*

I gloved up and cleaned Tim's wounds, which extended from his belly button to his tailbone. They were deep, and fluids oozed and dripped. His stomach was wide open, and I didn't want to put him in further pain. I didn't want to do any of it. I wanted to be his wife, his love. I never wanted to be the reason for any part of his pain.

It truly is astounding the things you have to do as a caregiver. This wasn't giving him medication and keeping him comfortable. This was a wake-up call.

Fortunately, the team at Memorial Sloan Kettering is amazing. It's because of them that Tim is still alive, six years and over thirty surgeries later. And they listen to us. For example, Tim and I have three basic rules, and they willingly comply.

Rule #1: Tim is one in a million. Statistics aren't something we're interested in hearing, and Tim is not a statistic.

Rule #2: We aren't doctors and, therefore, want to be spoken to in layman's terms.

Rule #3: Cancer isn't stealing one day of our life. We're not just living; we're living fully. So speak with optimism, and even better, throw in some humor if you feel compelled.

And my rule for caregiving is to meet Tim where he's at. If he wants to discuss, I am open and attentive. If he doesn't want to discuss, I am patient and understanding. Above all else, I shower him with unconditional love and remind him every single day that he's the love of my life.

At this point in our journey, I've gained confidence in my role as a caregiver. I don't have to swear, yell, or threaten anyone, but my words are pointed and firm. If you know deep down that something is amiss or altered, you need to speak up. You can't back down. Unfortunately, it took years to get to that point, and frankly, not everyone has that kind of time.

Tim's taken his story on the road, traveling the country performing a one-man comedy show: *The Shit Show. For real.* In his words, the show is a self-defecating one-man comedy show on how he battles cancer through humor, and his experiences facing chemo, radiation, a barrage of surgeries, home renovations, family, and puppies. A percentage of every ticket sold goes to a cancer organization in the city where he performs.

The Shit Show is one of many blessings we've experienced on the journey. We've met extraordinary people like Gail, who Tim met in the radiation waiting room. Gail was having radiation for breast cancer, so the top of her gown was off, and the bottom of his was off.

"I guess this is the pants off, tops optional room," he quipped as he looked over at her. At first, she gave him this look—but then she started to laugh and couldn't stop. We've had two Christmases and one Thanksgiving with Gail, her family, and friends. She's become our chosen family.

We've been the recipient of extraordinary generosity, too. People we've never even met gave us their Lexington Avenue apartment to use, complete with views of the Empire State Building. We stayed there for six weeks, then again for nearly three months during that crazy COVID-19 time. Tim's treatment required us to stay somewhere that had a kitchen and laundry, so we couldn't stay in hotels. One of our friends made an introduction to this couple, and they offered us the apartment, "It's yours whenever you need it." The kindness of strangers has been overwhelming.

The community in South Burlington, Vermont, has been amazing as well. Tim had done a lot of volunteering and MCing for nonprofits all over the state. He had his own game show and is very loved. After years of giving his time to the community, they have returned it tenfold. People drop off paper bags with eggs or maple syrup all the time. There's been a tremendous out-pouring of love and support by so many Vermonters.

Then there's Angel Flight Northeast, a nonprofit organization that pro-vides patients with flights to hospitals throughout the Northeast. Angel Flight was founded by Father Larry Camerlin twenty-six years ago and is run by a crew of some of the most generous people you'll ever meet. Heather is truly our angel at Angel Flight. The group of pilots, all of whom donate 100% of the costs, including their own time and private planes, are an exceptional group. We've taken nearly eighty flights with them from Burlington to New York City and call many of the pilot's friends at this point. They share our sorrows and our victories. They have literally extended Tim's life, and we can't say enough about them. Everyone should know about Angel Flight. What a true blessing.

And finally, the greatest blessing: my relationship with Tim. Six years, four cancer diagnoses, a permanent colostomy, and surgery every three months to repair past damages. I am so in awe of him and his amazing attitude.

We made an agreement early on that cancer would not steal the joy from our days or lives. Before I met Tim, I started a Joy Jar to demonstrate to my kids—and remind myself—of all the good there is in a year. It's hard to re-member when you're faced with so many challenges. Anytime something great happens, we write it down on a piece of paper with a date on it and put it in the Joy jar. Tim and I celebrate everything from all the ways we put smiles on each other's faces to the kindness of strangers to the magnitude of fun our kids, grandkids, family, and friends bring us. We see the jar every day but only read the notes on New Year's Day. We even find notes and little cartoons that others have left when they've visited us. The notes cover the table; tears spill from our eyes with laughter and the magic of memories.

Cancer has taken a lot of things from us. We never thought this was how our relationship would be, but one thing I know for certain is that cancer will not steal Tim's soul. There might be a day when we won't be together;

we don't talk about it, and we don't entertain it—because we're living in the present. We've made a choice to enjoy every minute together.

My caregiving journey with Tim has lifted me up and made me stronger. Sometimes people will say, "How sad you didn't meet sooner and could have had more time before all these cancer challenges." I think just the opposite. Tim and I came into each other's lives at just the right moment. God put us together knowing we can conquer anything. I admittedly wish Tim didn't have cancer, but I wouldn't change a thing. He's my love of life, and we're in this together, all the way.

 Candy Kavanagh lives with her husband Tim, and their rescue therapy dog, Adora, in South Burlington, Vermont. They have 5 children, 2 daughters-in-law and 2 grandchildren. She owns Weston Design, a full-service interior design firm. If cancer caregivers would like to contact Candy, her email is zencaregiver@yahoo.com.

MY TURN

by Bob Bennett

Who envisions a new, full-time career upon retiring at age seventy? I thought I would be doing a lot of trout fishing. I had another thing coming, courtesy of my bride of a similar age. She planned to retire from her job as office manager for a neurosurgeon, hoping to be a full-time grandmother of our first grandchild.

Not quite yet. She caught her shoe in a fax machine cord and broke her hip.

Over the next several years, she broke the other hip, suffered two strokes, and underwent a kidney operation, then another for skin cancer. And then there was an infected foot, a couple of UTIs, and some internal bleeding that put her in the hospital again. All this, in addition to rheumatoid arthritis.

I nearly wore the paint off the numbers 911 on our land line.

Now, she needs several pills a day, visiting nurses, physical therapy, two walkers (one for upstairs and one for down), a cane, stairlift, and two special chairs that help her to stand. She needs help to get out of bed and with everything in the bathroom, not to mention the unmentionables.

She needs help getting dressed. The last is the most challenging part of the day for yours truly—the would-be trout fisherman. She needs to be dressed in style, and I must display drawers full of sweaters and blouses and then hold up hanger after hanger of slacks for her approval. Socks must match.

So I cool my heels for excruciating minutes while she decides what to wear. And I do her hair.

I get the breakfast and take care of all the household duties this wonderful woman did for me for so many years—sixty-one now and counting. I'm a cook these days and getting better at it. In the evening, I put her on the stair-lift, into the bathroom again, into pajamas again, and into bed again.

What do I think about the situation? It's the best job I ever had, and I have had quite a few. It's my chance to help and be close to the woman who has done so much for me for so long. I wouldn't trade this job for anything. It's a privilege.

There are lots of rewards, but I think the best is getting special attention from her. I'm no longer playing second fiddle to our three kids, for whom she was a helicopter mother over the years. There's no greater satisfaction in my life than being able to help this wonderful woman.

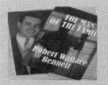

A resident of Vermont, Bob Bennett has published 10 nonfiction books, including his newest (under Robert Wallace Bennett) entitled, *The Man of the Family*. In 1942, a New Jersey boy's father leaves his wife and three boys "to kill Hitler." Before he goes, he tells the oldest, six, he is now "The Man of the Family." While WWII rages on, the family moves to Vermont, ostensibly to "spend the war," but the six-year-old is now 80 years older and still lives in the Green Mountain state. *The Man of the Family* follows him all those years as he attempts to live up to his father's charge and includes all its rejections and successes in love and business. You can find the book on Amazon.

PREPARING THE CAREGIVER

by Concetta Sullivan

Tears welled in my eyes as I read the email.

The message was from an old coworker. We hadn't spoken in years, and I just assumed she was contacting me to ask about being a job reference, but that wasn't the case.

I was so young when we first met. Fresh out of graduate school, I was well versed in anatomy, up-to-date on the latest research, and confident in my hands-on techniques—I was ready to become the best physical therapist for my patients. Of course, this was all theoretical or "paper knowledge;" this was my very first job as a physical therapist, under my own license, with real patients.

After a week of training with my mentor, I had my first physical therapy evaluation. As I had done so many times before in school, I read the patient's chart, which documented her broken leg from a fall down a flight of stairs. She was in the middle of a series of surgeries to reset the damaged leg bones, and she was in rehab to let the bones heal in the correct position so she could withstand her final surgery.

The orthopedic surgeon was keeping her bones together and in the correct position through external fixation (ex fix), which involved drilling the hardware from the outside of her body. I had only seen an ex fix in pictures, never in real life. As my stomach churned, I shuffled through the paperwork. I knew from my schooling that an ex fix typically corresponds with the weight-bearing status of nonbearing weight or NWB, so basically, the patient would not even be allowed to rest her foot on the ground.

The paperwork confirmed my suspicion: she was NWB on her lower left leg. I tried to keep a calm and collected face, as my mentor was watching my every move to ensure, above all else, that the patient received the best treatment from me, a very inexperienced physical therapist.

How am I going to help this poor woman walk again, I fretted.

The woman's whole ordeal started because she fell while walking up the stairs, and the orthopedic surgeon hadn't even scheduled her next surgery to remove the ex fix because her bones were still too brittle. And now she wasn't even allowed to place both feet on the ground?

What the hell am I supposed to do with her?

Although my mentor was right beside me, this was my first time running the show. I entered the rehab room of this eighty-eight-year-old woman and was greeted with a warm smile. With a cute Belgian accent, the patient introduced herself as Eva, and her calm and peaceful presence washed away my nerves.

I looked at the bed, and there was a massive bulge where Eva's leg should have been. And there it was, my first ex fix, still covered under a sheet. Before I could confront what lurked beneath the thin white sheet, I had to get to know Eva first. I sat with her and asked lots of questions, trying to pull together an extensive history of her life. While interviewing Eva, I realized that the flight of stairs that caused the fall would also prevent her from getting back into her apartment before the ex fix was explanted, and she was full weight-bearing. Until her bones healed up for her final surgery, Eva would be with us in the rehab facility.

Then it was time. It was time to see the ex fix, but more importantly, to see how her skin was healing up from the surgery. Slowly I pulled up the sheet covering Eva's leg and took in the structure holding her bones in place. Although Eva's leg was swollen, I realized that it wasn't all that gross. It looked like an erector set, drilled deep into the bones, allowing Eva's leg to have the blood supply it needed for proper healing.

At this point, my mentor stepped in to help me move the patient off the bed to prevent pneumonia and bedsores, and so that she could sit up to eat lunch safely. My mentor started rattling off the "rules for moving patients" with ex fixes.

Never grab in between the fixation. Above and below at the hip and ankle only. If you absolutely have to, you can grab a bar (part of the erector set), but never at the knee or anything in between the fixation.

Eva sat up on the edge of the bed, and with her change in position, blood began to pool in the affected extremity, causing her unimaginable pain. Eva screamed out. I quickly looked at my mentor for reassurance, fearing I had done something wrong.

Speaking to Eva and me in a calm voice, she said, "Because of gravity, it is normal to have pain when sitting on the edge of bed." My breathing slowed, and Eva matched my breaths. Soon, the pain subsided. Once Eva's composure returned, I asked her, "Do you still want to get to the chair today?"

Eva looked at me and said, "I'm feeling better, and I really want to eat lunch in my chair today. Please help me over there."

Together, and with the use of her walker, it took all of our combined strength to safely guide her over to the chair. Once Eva sat down, a big smile lit up her face; she was so excited to get to eat sitting upright while watching her favorite soap opera.

Eva and I spent an hour together every day to build up her strength, and after her final surgery, her weight-bearing status returned to full support. I got to know Eva well. Among all of the stories we swapped while Eva took rest breaks in the hallway, my favorite was when I asked Eva about her thumb ring. With a smile, Eva explained it was her late husband's wedding band; she referred to herself as a "war bride of World War II."

While Eva worked hard on building her strength and safety while walking on her own, I worked hard building my confidence and applying physical therapy skills to my real-world patients. With each patient, I developed this unique bond—one that only a therapist and a patient can really know.

The day came when Eva was finally able to walk up the flight of stairs in the gym safely, thanks to all of the hard work we had both put in over the previous months. It was time to start the discharge planning. I had never met Eva's family prior to their caregiving training, but we went over a comprehensive plan to keep Eva safe. Things like how to safely guard her on the stairs so she wouldn't lose her balance and fall again, removing any trip hazards in Eva's house, like throw rugs, and even adding night lights, among many other suggestions. They listened intently and took notes. I could tell that her caregivers were going to do an amazing job helping Eva do what she wanted to do the most—get back to living in her own home.

I said goodbye to Eva, but not before telling her how proud I was of her. She really put the work in, and I was thrilled that she was headed home. And then, just like any other day, I went on to see my next patient.

Ten years later, I received an email from my former mentor, sharing the news that Eva had passed peacefully in her home, surrounded by the caregivers who listened so attentively upon her discharge from my care—her family.

Caregiving often begins in the hospital or rehabilitation facilities. We don't always think about it, but it's an essential part of the journey. Especially nowadays, when families are asked to take on complicated caregiving tasks, things that go well beyond the basics: food, clothing, bathing, and safety. Before your loved one is discharged, make sure you understand what is being asked of you. Ask a lot of questions and know that you are not being insecure or weak. It's our job to make sure you have the information, and sometimes, the skills to be an effective caregiver.

The caregiving journey may start with doctors, nurses, and therapists, but once you get home, the greatest burden and greatest blessing—caregiving—shifts to you and your family.

Concetta Sullivan received her Doctor of Physical Therapy from Simmons University in 2013. Since then, she has worked in many different settings with a wide variety of patients, each of them teaching her a lesson. She currently specializes in pelvic floor physical therapy. Recently Concetta has entered the world of writing, which allows her to share these lessons with a broader audience through a fictional setting.

SOMETHING BIG

by Tony Stoddard

Sixteen years ago, my wife and I received the most amazing news. *We were going to have twins.* Our daughter Tara was three years old at the time, and we had been trying for quite a while to have another child, but twins? We were shocked, nervous, and excited about the future of our family.

Our twin boys, Cole, and Troy, were born in 2006. They were born premature and spent a month in incubators as their frail bodies struggled to grow bigger and stronger. The day we were finally able to bring them home was joyous, but as we soon learned, it was demanding and exhausting, too. Being the caretakers of one child was hard enough, but taking care of our young daughter and now two infant boys was a monumental task.

Many sleepless nights and emotionally and physically demanding days were to come. At the time, I thought nothing could be harder than taking care of our three children while working and managing daily life. Four short years later, things got harder—much harder.

I had been taking Troy and Cole to a nearby athletic club for swimming lessons a few days each week. They loved to swim, and it made me so happy to see my boys enjoying themselves. One day, they both woke up complaining of earaches, and they also had fevers. We brought them to our pediatrician, and they were diagnosed with ear infections, possibly caused by the pool water in which they had been swimming.

Cole and Troy were prescribed antibiotics to clear the infections. Troy responded well to the medication and began to feel better after a couple of days, but his identical twin brother Cole only got sicker.

Their doctor recommended that Cole have an X-ray of his chest; she feared that he may have developed pneumonia. My wife, Michelle, brought Cole for the X-ray while I stayed home with our other two children, anxiously awaiting the results. Soon after, my wife called and asked me to bring Troy and Tara to my sister-in-law's house; she said she needed to talk to me alone.

Immediately, I knew something was terribly wrong. When Michelle returned home, she told me the X-rays showed an orange-sized mass behind one of Cole's kidneys—a mass that was most likely cancer. I went into our bedroom and screamed into a pillow, "No, No, No!" over and over again until I had no voice left to scream.

That night, my wife took Cole to the Tufts Floating Hospital for Children in Boston, Massachusetts for further tests while I once again stayed home to be with Troy and Tara. When I arrived at the hospital the next day, we met with a team of doctors who informed us that Cole had neuroblastoma cancer and that his odds of survival were about thirty-five percent. Michelle broke down in tears, and I tried my best to reassure her that Cole would beat this disease. I genuinely believed that through miracles or medicine, Cole would be okay. *He had to be.*

Multiple surgeries, radiation treatments, and rounds of chemotherapy began. It tore my soul to bits to watch my son suffer so deeply. My wife was so incredibly strong throughout the year and a half that Cole battled cancer. She somehow found the strength to stay organized—scheduling appointments, keeping track of Cole's medications and procedures, and ensuring Troy and Tara lived as normally as possible each day.

Honestly, I don't know how she did it. I found that my role as a caretaker during this horrific situation was to simply be a silly dad, focused on helping my kids smile and laugh, playing with them, and fighting to have Cole at home as much as possible to be with the ones he loved.

Michelle and I were so afraid of what lay ahead and how we would get through this painful place in our lives, but quickly, we were showered with the most extraordinary display of love and support from family, friends, neighbors, work colleagues, former classmates, and even numerous strangers. We have a very close-knit family, and they all took turns watching Troy and Tara when we were at the hospital during Cole's treatments. Our community organized to provide us with meals and household supplies, gift cards, and much more so that we could focus on trying to get Cole better.

Because we both missed so much work, family members and friends created fundraising events to help, and organizations and individuals provided us with financial support to help alleviate monetary worries. A family friend, who owns a facility called Hampstead Health and Fitness, invited us to use his gym at any time. Keeping my body stronger also helped me remain stronger mentally so that I didn't completely fall apart. In our darkest time, individuals rallied around us to help bring a glimmer of light.

School children from many districts around us sent Cole, Troy, and Tara hundreds of letters of hope and love. Each day, gifts and toys were delivered to our home to help bring some cheer to our children. The outpouring of caring was truly astounding and will always be profoundly appreciated and never forgotten.

As the cancer in Cole's body continued to spread, daily life became even more difficult. There were times when we needed to wake Cole up every hour to take his medications. My wife and I were constantly bordering on the edge of complete exhaustion. None of Cole's treatments had done anything to fight the cancer, and Cole became weaker and in deeper pain. Each time our boy finished a round of chemo, the follow-up scans showed that there was no positive effect on the cancer. The monster in my son's body continued to multiply.

Still, we refused to give up hope, seeking second, third, and fourth opinions from oncologists across the world. I prayed every day for God to take the cancer from Cole and give it to me a thousand times worse, if that was what it would take to ease my son's agony.

There was one time when Cole received a Clinical Trial that showed a glimmer of promise. Cole received MIBG Therapy, which bombards the cells with radiation designed to kill the cancer cells. To receive this therapy, Cole had to be isolated in a small lead-enclosed room for a week. Only one parent was allowed to stay with him during this time.

Michelle stayed with Cole during this harsh treatment, as she is more capable of staying calm and reassuring under stress than I am. It was better for Cole to be with his mom at these times. Her ability to smile through the pain and to give comfort in the most trying of situations is something I admire more than I can express.

After this therapy, scans showed that there was some decrease in cancer cells. Finally, we had found something that showed an ounce of promise. Cole's doctors immediately scheduled another round of MIBG, hoping that it would continue to work. However, after the second round of radiation, the cancer cells had actually increased. Our hope was shattered. I think at this moment. we began to accept that we had run out of options and that it was time to refocus on simply keeping Cole as comfortable as possible and alleviating his pain as best we could.

The Make-A-Wish Foundation of New Hampshire came into our lives at this point and allowed our family to spend a magical week at Disney World in Florida, creating many cherished memories. We still hoped for a miracle, but in reality, we were simply trying to make as many happy memories as possible.

In December of 2011, Cole was worn down. His doctors had advised us that they had done all that they could. We spent countless hours at his bedside, placing heating pads on the areas of his frail body that were hurting him, singing songs to him, and gently caressing him. Cole was so heavily medicated that he slept most of each day. The tumors in his mouth made it difficult to speak, and he was basically immobile.

There was one miraculous moment when my wife and I sat quietly beside Cole's hospital bed when suddenly, he raised his head from his pillow and said, "Smile, be happy." He began to lower his head but rose up once again, then more forcefully said, "Smile, be happy!" We were stunned. We believe that Cole knew we would hurt for the rest of our lives when he was gone and that he wanted—no, demanded—that we find ways to laugh, smile, and find happiness in the time we had left in this life.

That was Cole's wish for us all—that was Cole's lasting gift to us.

Shortly before Cole died, I was lying next to him in his bed watching television. When a police officer appeared on the show we were viewing, I asked Cole if he still wanted to be a policeman or firefighter when he grew up—Cole idolized first responders—but he quietly replied that he wouldn't grow up to be anything. Hearing my son say, and know, that he would not grow up broke my heart.

Fighting back tears, I promised him he would do "something big" someday. He asked what that would be. I told him, "I don't really know right now, but I promise you will do something big, something important." Cole seemed satisfied with this reply.

Cole passed away on January 20, 2012, at age five. I honestly did not think I would be able to survive losing him, but I had two other children who still needed me, and I had my promise to Cole to keep. Months later, when my mind began to clear somewhat from the excruciating grief I was mired in, it suddenly hit me what Cole's "something big" would be.

It was midway through September, which is Childhood Cancer Awareness Month. My wife and I were working together on a fundraiser for childhood cancer research when a commercial came on TV for Breast Cancer Awareness. My wife and I stopped what we were doing and both had the same thought. We needed to do everything we could to make September's Childhood Cancer Awareness Month as widespread as October's Breast Cancer Awareness Month was—in Cole's memory.

We both knew that in order for childhood cancer research funding to increase, we needed to make others aware of the fact that childhood cancer is the number one killer disease of kids in our country, and that funding to research cures for it and finding more humane treatments for our children affected by cancer needed to begin with greater awareness. After all, "How can you expect people to care, unless you first make them aware."

I immediately began contacting officials who displayed pink in October at major buildings, bridges, landmarks, and sports facilities, asking if they would also light gold in September for kids battling cancer. Almost everyone I reached out to agreed to do so. Iconic structures such as the Prudential Tower and the Zakim Bridge in Boston began to light gold in September. When the media reported on these displays of gold and the reason behind it, many other monuments soon followed in lighting gold to help raise childhood cancer awareness. Others in the childhood cancer community soon joined in this effort, and with their influence, gold began to spread across the world in September. Today, even Major League Baseball and the White House now light gold in September in honor of all children battling cancer and in memory of those who sadly were taken from us by this disease.

Fighting for greater awareness and funding for children affected by cancer gave me something big to live for, and it brought me peace that I had kept my promise to Cole.

A few years after Cole passed away, he sent me a sign that he wanted me to thru-hike the Appalachian Trail as a way to help in this endeavor. I made it about five hundred miles across this difficult trek before I sustained a serious knee injury. I was demoralized that I wasn't able to finish all 2,200 miles of the trail, but I was determined to heal and finish the trail the next year. However, a month before I planned to return to where I left off, I, too, was diagnosed with cancer.

I had been having stomach issues, and it was recommended that I have a colonoscopy. This procedure indicated that I had tumors in my colon. On hearing my doctor say that I had stage 3 colon cancer, my first thought was, I can't believe I'm going to put my kids through the pain of having a family member deal with cancer once again. My next thought was, *How can I use my cancer to help kids battling this monster?*

Friends, family, and community members came to our rescue once more, providing us with financial assistance, love, and moral support as I fought to survive. It sounds strange to say this as a family that has lost a child to cancer and also having it strike in my body, but we are truly blessed. Caretakers surrounded us everywhere. Through the goodness that is all around, we have been able to endure as a family, and we have even been able to fulfill Cole's wish that we always do our best to smile and be happy!

There are heartbreakers, and there are caretakers in this world. Please always choose to be a caretaker and spread love and joy whenever possible, and if you are suffering and in need, remember that the best way to heal is to heal someone else.

Tony Stoddard is a father, husband, son, and friend. He's also a cancer survivor, keeper of promises, and a fierce childhood cancer advocate.

HOW TO KEEP GOING

by Dave Cantillon

There are countless angles to being a caregiver. Over the years, I've been party to a number of serious tragedies. As a teenager, my older sister was in a terrible house fire leaving her badly scarred with a quarter of her body sustaining third-degree burns. I would accompany my mother to the hospital for many visits, and through many reconstructive surgeries, I saw my sister persevere during the difficult years to follow.

Many years later, after several years of marriage, my wife and I became the parents of our only child, Ben, with Down syndrome and Hirschsprung's disease. The latter is a defect of the large intestine, or colon, that processes waste by moving it as it travels for eventual discharge. Nerve cells in the colon are defective, so they don't fire to facilitate passage, which results in obstruction.

In the first few years of his life, he needed numerous surgeries in order to survive. A colostomy bag as a baby, later reconnected only to have the colostomy bag back again. Surgeons repaired his rectum, which had painful fissures. His entire colon was removed. The small intestine was surgically attached to his rectum and anus, ending the need for the colostomy, but because the colon extracts moisture, his discharge was more of a liquid. The repair of his fissures resulted in the loss of full control.

Ben turned twenty in 2022, is nonverbal, still in diapers, and on the low end of cognitive function. He has a pleasant disposition and is a joy to us. He also uses some sign language and has completed his schooling.

The description you just read is misleading because you might picture a boatload of unpleasantness. To be clear, he has some control. However, his cognitive and nonverbal challenges have taken us down a road over the years where we've learned to schedule his daily life, and ours, around his needs—

and continue to help him acquire life skills for managing himself. We take walks around the block. He loves his iPad and plays games and music, enjoys a PC in his bedroom, and enjoys pizza like most of us. He's learned to sign his name and helps dress himself, but he still struggles with other tasks.

We love him. He loves us. We are a happy family with a handicapped child.

We know very well what caregiving entails and admire those families and individuals who are sacrificing themselves to care for a loved one. Our personal challenges are different. We've learned to roll with the punches. He's had a total of fourteen surgeries and almost died as a baby. Like many caregivers, my wife and I try to see the humor in the day-to-day struggles and navigate the frustrations to the best of our ability. We view life as sacred and love our son. We've learned to accept that many who know us will never quite understand what we've been through. There are days when shades of resentment will bubble up.

For example, in conversation, someone will ask how he's doing at school and proceed to share some accomplishments of their own children. Something like this: "Our Johnny did so well, counselors are recommending we apply for some scholarships!"

We're happy for their son, but ours was incapable of taking standard tests, won't hold a crayon properly or color within lines, and spends a great deal of time on the potty. Not that we're competing, yet such conversations just remind us of how far behind and extraordinary our son is. Some of the support groups we've joined to help us have been a source of tremendous encouragement. You know *they* understand. They're dealing with it as well. There is strength to be drawn from others who persevere.

They know the struggle. They know the routines. They appreciate the swings between diligence and exhaustion.

Caregiving has a life of its own, so to speak. There are days when you spring out of bed ready to address anything that comes up, whistling through whatever trial presents itself. Although our son may not show appreciation, we know in our hearts that we've really done our best and are confident he feels loved and cared for. Those are good days.

The others swing into a lower realm of depleted energy and defeat. We continue to work through the routines, but there isn't a feeling of accomplishment. It's drudgery. We're content to just stare at the TV, glad to do nothing. If a chore can wait, it does. Forget dinner. We'll eat cereal. On the weak days, a sense of guilt comes in and out with the same persistent message: "You're not doing enough." To which a host of excuses flow. From I've-done-enough-already to I'm-not-in-the-mood-to-care.

Inevitably, the work presents itself again, and you do what has to be done. For our son, it's changing his diapers, changing the bed, checking for sores, and ensuring he's safe and occupied.

On the weak days, there's a sense of being trapped. As an example, suppose you have a taste for a Mexican dish and start thinking about going to a restaurant. We can't just jump up and go. We look at the clock, and the routines kick in.

Has he gone potty? When did he last go? When does he need to be put back on? If we bring him to the restaurant, do we have his diaper bag? Is it packed with everything? Ointments, pads, rubber pants and a change of clothes (in case he leaks).

Then you assess the risks involved. What if he has an accident? It's one thing to change a baby in a restaurant's restroom, but when you're dealing with an adult-sized young man, the size of the stall becomes an issue. And the waiting? What if there's a wait? The cleanliness of the floor. Other customers coming in and out.

In other words, you can't really be spontaneous. Everything has to be planned and readied. On a good day, we get everything in order and have a nice outing. On the bad days, we make a sandwich or cook a frozen pizza. In other words, you have a taste for Mexican, but you don't have the stamina for the routine. And if you're in that frustrated mood, you feel trapped, prohibited from enjoying life.

On strong days, there are many joys. We note progress. He'll do something we hadn't anticipated. He'll put socks away in a drawer when we weren't at first even sure he knew where his socks go. He'll take off his shirt and put on a different one all on his own. It might be backward, but for us, it's a joy because he's deliberate and learning. We hug him a lot, and he hugs us back. He'll be laughing out loud at something he's watching on his iPad. He'll verbalize at long stretches as if he's talking to himself. Although we don't understand what he's saying, we're confident it's meaningful, and we'll call from the other room, "I know what you mean!" He'll cooperate. He'll show appreciation by squeezing our arm as if to be telling us he appreciates what we're doing for him.

Going to bed is always a genuine pleasure. He's a great sleeper, so when it's time to retire, he'll be glad to be tucked in, made comfortable, and quickly falls asleep. It's not so hard to describe, but any caregiver would agree. When everything is done and the day is done, it's a rewarding feeling.

Let life come at me tomorrow. For now, I can just let go.

Another aspect of caregiving is the education you receive. Medically, you acquire the terms and language of the circumstance. You pick up some of the lingo in hospitals. You acquire knowledge of medical products—their purpose, their utility. You learn about distinctions. For example, instead of resorting to the outdated term "retarded" (which is now considered offensive), we use terms like "developmentally disabled" or "cognitively delayed." Instead of saying "stupid," we say "slow."

These are the kinds of shifts in language you navigate. It's funny, but on some days when you've got the caregiving cape on and feel resilient to the general lack of awareness many show, you may be inclined to jump to advocacy. Some shoppers will look at the way a product is packaged and shout, "Oh my! This is so retarded!" and we'll wince. Maybe call them out on it, if the atmosphere allows for it. In a conversation, someone will complain about some errant behavior observed and what a ridiculous scene that unfolded. We'll respond by offering another point of view, that maybe there was a sensory issue involved or a hidden disability not appreciated—almost insinuating that the gripe was not only inappropriate but rude, or worse, insensitive and degrading to the unfortunate.

All this comes with the territory.

Over the years, caregiving has been a journey with hills and valleys. On rare occasions, someone might open up and genuinely want to know what we've been doing. We'll start to unpack and unload the many details of caring for our son. The brushing of the teeth, the trimming of the nails, the braces on his feet, the changing of the diapers, the scheduling of the potty, the worry of his sickness, the danger he can be to himself, the longing to anticipate speech, the frustration of now knowing what he's asking for, and the tools we use to communicate what we can. It's overwhelming. There are so many things to know, watch for, and be cautious about. His glasses. His shoes. Not just the diaper but the tabs on the diapers, the condition of the pull ups that go over the diaper, and the condition of the rubber pants that go over the pull-ups.

My wife and I always appreciate the compassion shown to us. Our faith has kept us strong. We have both family and friends who have been very supportive. We don't like asking for help but appreciate when it's offered. The journey has involved a boat load of professionals that have helped us navigate all the complexity of his education, the support, and programs available to him, the medical procedures necessary for his health, and ongoing care for things that come up, including dental work and skin abrasions and boils.

I suppose writing about caregiving would be comparable to writing about swimming. You can describe water. You can describe splashing, describe holding your breath, different strokes, and how to get water out of your ear. But to really appreciate swimming, you have to jump in the water and see for yourself. Then you'll know. So, in the case of caregiving, I'll add to the depth of your appreciation by sharing a few events in our journey.

We have to laugh about it. We don't want to cry and buckle. We take it in stride and try to see humor in it. We're glad when bad days pass and keep that noxious, overwhelming fear at bay as we take it on day by day. For the rest of this piece, I'll tell you things that have happened.

The Mustard Pack

When Ben was a little over one, he had to have a colostomy bag to allow his rectum to heal enough for a later procedure. One of our friends offered to bring us Chinese takeout while Ben was recovering. We were also given a little stuffed figure of Piglet from *Winnie the Pooh*, which lay by his side, about four or five inches tall. The mustard pack that came with the egg rolls was comparable to the color of the contents of his recovery colostomy bag. I grabbed some surgical tape in the room and taped the mustard pack to the side of Piglet and made it look like Piglet had a colostomy bag, just like my son.

When the surgeon came in for his rounds to check on Ben, he roared with laughter.

The Rain

Ben had to have multiple surgeries for his colon and rectum when they attached his small intestine to his rectum. During one of the attachments, he was wheeled from surgery to his room for monitoring while he healed. He had a catheter inserted to take care of his bladder. After the first hour, the nurse came in to check his bag to see if he was producing urine.

That was a worry. She notified surgery. They advised her to keep monitoring, as Ben was still coming off of anesthesia. Another hour passed, and still no urine. This was now a problem.

The hospital was a teaching hospital, and the surgeon sent two interns to our room to examine him. His belly was still soft, and he appeared comfortable. They reported back to the surgeon and advised to continue monitoring for another hour. Still nothing. This time, his nurse was instructed to check the catheter. A blocked catheter is rare, even highly unlikely. She said they hardly ever pull a catheter once it's been inserted post-surgery and that would be very unusual, but he really needed to show output, and so there we were.

My wife and I, my mother-in-law, and the nurse at the bedside were worried he might need an emergency surgical intervention for his bladder.

She held up his little dinky, smaller than a thimble, and gently pulled the catheter. It's not every day you appreciate being urinated on, but we all rejoiced as the flood gates opened and arched on all of us before we quickly grabbed a diaper to absorb the flood.

Immunity

One of the ongoing challenges with Ben was his susceptibility to infections. One of the functions of the large intestine is to absorb water. Without one, it became critically important to always keep Ben hydrated, especially if he was sick from any kind of food. He could quickly dehydrate. Several times we had to take him to an emergency room for some help getting him rehydrated with an IV.

To make matters worse, he was always licking things and touching things and showing no regard for hygiene. He was a big drooler, and we had to buy plastic tubes for him to chew on as he was growing because he thrived on having something in his mouth. We kept a rag handy all the time to keep his face and chin dry as he aged. If he was near a door, he would lick the wood. If you put a pen on the table, he would feel it and lick it. We were always cautious about change and money, knowing how frequently handled it is.

One winter day when Ben was about four, I wanted him to get some exercise. He wasn't a great walker and needed special braces. I didn't want him to be outside, but I felt a nice walk would do him good. I took him to the airport, where he could ride the escalators, walk between terminals, and get some decent walking in. There was a long moving sidewalk stretching between domestic and international travelers; you could call it a flat escalator with railings and all. He was thrilled to move along and enjoy the "ride," and I was proud to help him.

I looked down to check on him and discovered he was licking the *handrail. International germs.* In my heart, I was ready to incur yet another deductible on his health insurance. *Yikes.*

The Stick

On another occasion, our son contracted some kind of bug, which we were trying to manage with electrolytes in a sports drink hoping to avoid a trip to the ER. Give him that boost to avoid dehydration. Because he hadn't learned how to drink out of a glass, we presented him with a plastic cup with a straw. Not feeling well, he refused to drink even when we encouraged him to do so. This resistance was part of the cognitive disability related to behavior and communication. Mind you, he was older, around ten, and getting stronger as a boy, but his health deteriorated rapidly, and we couldn't keep up with the fever. We were even using syringes filled with Gatorade and trying to squirt it into his mouth, which he fought.

By now, we were well aware of his need for hydration. This is one of the side effects of Hirschsprung's and Down syndrome combined. We packed him up and headed to the ER knowing we could explain that his need for an IV to boost his hydration. Parents end up knowing these things intuitively, and we learned it from Ben. It was just a bug, and he needed support. An intern working in the ER understood all we explained and ordered a blood draw just to confirm. We ended up being right and were sent home after many hours of this intervention.

Getting the blood for the blood test, however, was the adventure here. The dehydration and his skin tone and flabbiness made it difficult for the nurse to find a vein. Stick #1: It was handled all so fast he barely had time to react, but unsuccessful. Stick #2: Now he's wise to what's happening, pulling his arm away and fighting the nurse while my wife and I are holding him down. Stick #3: Two nurses come in and help us hold him down while he's sweating, fighting us with all his might. Stick #4: A special nurse from the "IV Team" was paged to assist and attempted another spot with four of us holding him down, and now he's screaming. He's sweating. We're drained. The nurses are baffled.

Finally, the head doctor on call was pulled from whatever he was doing to assist. We knew we were up for another fight, so another staff member came in to help keep him still. We practically had to sit on him. The doctor was able to find a channel and succeeded in establishing the draw and a port for the hydration. That was stick #5.

As we held him down, the doctor asked for some alcohol wipes for the area, and the nurse had already exhausted her pockets and reached for a cabinet in the room, which was under lock and key and could only be opened with a designated swipe of a special card. She was holding one of his limbs, and the rest of us had him pinned, the doctor on the other side.

Imagine the scene. Six people in the room struggling to complete this draw and stick, one of them stretching sidewise to reach with her card to unlock the cabinet for a simple alcohol wipe, one hand on his limb, the other trying to reach the cabinet. They all assured us this was highly unusual. This was a children's hospital. It was surreal, yet we had come to understand that our son often presented atypical health problems associated with Down syndrome.

It all worked out, but what an episode. He was a regular pin cushion that night.

The Meeting

When Ben started in a different school building beyond the initial program for Down syndrome children, we quickly learned that the classroom he was in wasn't set up to accommodate his diapering accidents. His missing colon meant that the fluidity of his discharge often leaked beyond his diaper and soiled classroom materials being used by other children. The room he was assigned to did not have an adjoining bathroom, and trips down the hall were problematic as well.

Thus began the routine, beginning with a phone call, "Please come get your son." Months went by with frequent requests to the point where his education was being compromised. We sought advice and were helped by school district representatives, a state parent mentor advocating for special needs, another agency advocating for the disabled, and legal counsel for the school district to address the failures. Imagine a conference room with eight people around the table to discuss my son's education.

To start the meeting, each person present was asked to introduce themselves. The Principal, the Advocate, the state official, the counsel . . . and when it got to me as Ben's dad, I said, "If you had told me when my son was born that one day, I would be sitting around a conference table with a bunch of professionals to discuss my son's crap, I wouldn't have believed it." That got the round of laughter it deserved, and Ben was transferred to a different school with a classroom that had an adjoining bathroom.

The Flush

During the periods when Ben had his colostomy bag, it was pretty stressful to change the wafer around his stomach. We had to keep things clean, and it was often stressful. We were visiting family in West Virginia and stayed at a local hotel, which provided a small pen for him at night. In the morning, I noted Ben's bag was puffy, which meant it needed emptying. We had purchased a foldable toilet seat, which rested on top of any toilet to support him while we emptied the bag. It fit nicely over the seat, and the bag was emptied successfully. I was supporting him with my left hand and reached momentarily for some tissue to clean the end of the bag when the foldable seat collapsed and landed my poor son sitting in the cold toilet water, his legs sticking out of the toilet. He was sucking on a binky and practically inhaled the thing. It was such a shock. I lifted him out of the toilet in his now soaking and soiled "onesie" and laid him on a towel and proceeded to clean him up thoroughly. As the story goes, we recall this treasured trip as the one we almost flushed our son down the toilet.

These are just a few of the incidents of being a caregiver. I almost hate to use the well-worn metaphor of peaks and valleys, but the daily dilemmas of caring for the kinds of challenges we've had taught us to expect anything. It's funny whenever we have to take him for a new medical procedure or for an exam, and the standard office form would state, "List medical history here," then give us about three lines. We would note a few of his conditions and then explain, but just reading that invoked an exhausting recall and the thought, "I'm gonna need more paper."

Ben's medical journey has made us resilient. We have learned to have compassion for anyone navigating special needs problems with a child, or for that matter, anyone who is caregiving. There have been several times over the years when we've approached families clearly struggling and have taken the time to introduce ourselves and offer encouragement. You wish you could give time and money, but even a few words would mean a lot to caregivers in a world where many just don't understand the weight of caregiving.

The power of love enables you to deliver. Oddly, it even enables you to forgive those who can't because we've learned that it really can be overwhelming. Some just don't have the stamina, and being a judge doesn't help. We are cheerleaders. We are compassionate. We are also weak. We often fail. In the face of enormous complexity and circumstances beyond our control, we do the best we can. Caregiving isn't an art. It's a mixture of duty and love. Our hope is always that by example, somehow, even when no one can see behind the walls of our home, we show those fearful of it, that things really can get done.

Life is a gift. Caregiving has its rewards. And although we wouldn't wish our circumstances on anyone, neither would we deny that it has taught us lessons we would never have learned otherwise.

Especially how to love, how to muster up strength, and how to keep going.

Husband, father, accounting professional and Minister, Dave Cantillon resides in Cleveland, OH.

THE GIRL REALLY LOVES ME

by Judy Peterson

I became a nurse by accident. I never had a strong "caregiving" instinct. Because I did well in science classes, my high school Guidance Counselor suggested that I become a nurse. I said "okay."

I joined the Peace Corps immediately after graduating from college, and in Central America, I fell in love with public health and community-based nursing care. After my return to the US, I enjoyed being a home health nurse for many years. I always loved teaching people about health maintenance and nutrition, but I never wanted to be a bedside nurse for critically ill people in the hospital.

Fast forward about ten years, and I met my soulmate, Ron. His history of dyslexia, recovery from alcoholism, and divorce after thirteen years of marriage had made him the kindest, most patient, and empathetic man I have ever known. I fell in love with him on our first date.

Years later, at the age of fifty-six, Ron contracted a virus that attacked his heart and left him with cardiomyopathy, a progressive weakening of the heart muscle, eventually leading to death. He was never able to work again after that virus attack, and we had two children in elementary school, so finances and everyday family and household duties became a considerable worry for us both. I increased my hours at work from 3/4 time to full time—which soon became fifty hours since I was salaried—and Ron took on non-strenuous activities like kid transportation, laundry, and generally being the "at home" presence for the kids. There were many days that I felt overworked and overwhelmed, but Ron and I could always talk about what we felt, and that was what kept us both afloat.

Ron lived for eight years after becoming ill. In the initial years, my caregiving experience was that of simply taking greater responsibility for what felt like "everything." That "everything" was related to daily family living and home maintenance. Much of my caregiving for Ron involved managing his medications and encouraging him to follow the doctor's orders regarding diet and exercise, as well as ensuring he attended necessary medical appointments and asked the doctor the right questions.

But there was another very important piece to it too. I always felt like I wanted Ron to still feel like the head of the household and the worthwhile and able human being he still was. Ron had been an electrician, an antique dealer, a hunter, an active father, a fun and energetic person, and an empathetic and capable sponsor for new members of AA. Now, there was so much he couldn't do. So I needed to capitalize on what he could do and let him know how helpful and important that was to our family.

Maybe he couldn't stack the wood, vacuum, or mow the lawn anymore, but he could drive the car to pick up kids, peel potatoes for dinner, fold the laundry, etc. He made my long work hours easier to accomplish because he held the fort at home, and I let him know how meaningful that was to me and the kids.

We took some lovely vacations during those eight years. Ron, and often the kids too, accompanied me on work trips for conferences. We attended several reunions with my old Peace Corps friends, and we always rented a camp on Groton Pond for a week in the summer. We lived life and enjoyed doing all the things a healthy family does. We just did it all a little slower—the kids and I did the heavy lifting, and we adjusted activities to make them manageable for everyone.

Ron's cardiomyopathy progressed slowly but surely, as there is no cure. He took lots of meds, which were changed when needed and managed well by our cardiologist. There were multiple hospitalizations, and he even had open heart surgery to replace a damaged valve, but there was no real improvement. There was just maintaining the status quo or slowing the weakening of his heart muscle. We explored a heart transplant, but he was not eligible since he was immunocompromised because of a previous bladder cancer that had returned.

Honestly, I think on some level we were both in denial about what the outcome would be. When Ron had one more crisis and hospitalization in October 2007, the cardiologist suggested we consider hospice admission. It was at that moment that we both suddenly remembered that in the ER that first night when he was diagnosed with cardiomyopathy, the doctors had told us he would have eight to ten years to live. We had conveniently forgotten, or perhaps buried, that piece of information. Now it came rushing into full view.

Ron lived six more weeks after that October hospitalization. He was home, and I was his primary caregiver. Both kids were in college, and I had just received a promotion at work, which required even longer work hours. I explained that I needed to work part-time, and my employer was very understanding. But of course—I felt guilty. Guilty for not being at home full time and guilty for not being at work full time. We had hospice nurses visit weekly for symptom management, an aide three times a week to help with a shower, and wonderful friends and family providing respite to fill the gaps when I was at work.

At that point, about a month before Ron died, I heard from a dear old friend in NY asking if she could come to help. At first, I said, " No, we're fine," but she gently asked how I was doing myself. Then I realized how stressed and overwhelmed I was, and I knew I couldn't take care of Ron the way I wanted to in that state. So, I said, "Yes. When can you be here?"

Brenda stayed for two weeks and was an amazing help. My decision to let her help us was difficult but was one of the most important decisions I made in those last weeks. I realized that to care for Ron, I had to also care for myself. I worked less during Brenda's two-week stay and then I didn't work at all during the last two weeks of Ron's life. Another friend came for a week—I was getting the hang of this "accepting help" thing—and she also did the meals and the cleaning and the errands, etc., as Brenda had.

All I did was spend time with Ron. We talked about his will, his memorial service, his burial, his regrets, his successes, his faith, and his hopes and dreams for our kids. It was wonderful, and I'll never forget this gift my friends gave me.

Both kids came home from college to spend the last week with their father. As a family, we laughed, we reminisced, and we cried. Our friends and relatives left, at my request. This was time for just us. Just the Peterson family.

At night, I slept on a mattress on the floor next to Ron's hospital bed that was set up in the living room so I would know if he needed anything. I woke up one morning with him looking at me with a slight smile on his lips. He said very quietly, in an almost whisper, "Well, I guess the girl really loves me." And he was right.

RELYING ON THE CAREGIVER

by Eileen Curran

My husband, Bob, doesn't remember much about the day he had his brain aneurysm. That's the thing about a traumatic brain injury; the person who experiences it remembers little if nothing about the event or the aftermath, but the people closest to them remember everything—every thought, feeling, emotion, and heartbeat. Every chaotic moment—along with the quiet ones, alone in the hospital chapel.

I had just arrived at a local salon for a quick appointment when I saw on my phone my husband was calling me. Knowing this would be a quick fifteen-minute appointment, I declined the call, intending to call him back when I got out. After the appointment, I checked my phone, and there were more calls from my husband and our daughter—I knew this wasn't good.

I called my husband first, and he answered the phone. He told me he had driven off the road and was being put into an ambulance. He then said something about the EMTs saying it was a stroke. I told myself to stay calm and ask questions. I asked Bob where they were taking him. He then repeated that he had gone off the road, and some people stopped, called 911, and gave him some really cold water. I again asked where the ambulance was taking him. He said he didn't know, so I said, "Please ask the EMT." The EMT gave the name of the hospital. I said I'm getting in my car and will meet you there.

On the way to the hospital, I called our teenage daughter, Grace. Our middle son, Dan, answered her phone. He said the police had called Grace and said they were taking Dad to the hospital. He told me they were getting in the car and heading there.

Then I called my friend Sue, who is a nurse at Massachusetts General Hospital and with whom we happened to have dinner plans that evening. I told her what happened. I asked if she knew any neurologists at MGH because

I was going to have Bob moved from our wonderful but small community hospital into Boston. She said she and her husband would meet us at the hospital.

To this day, people have asked me how I could be so calm while making phone calls and plans while driving to the hospital where my husband, who may have had a stroke, was being transported. Two things. First, he was able to speak to me on the phone, so I knew he was conscious, and that was a promising sign. And the other: I had spent many years as a news reporter covering stories of tragedies, fatal fires, murdered children, and 9/11.

News reporters can't respond to the scene of a tragedy and react with emotion. If you do, you won't be able to do your job. Instead, you compartmentalize and put your feelings in a box and go do your job. Once the story is done and you are driving home, you pull down that box and feel those feelings—as a wife, a mother, and a human being.

When I got to the hospital, the kids were in the waiting room, as well as my friend Sue and her husband, Rich. I told the kids that Dad was going to be alright, and for some unknown reason, I truly felt he would be.

The nurse let me go into his room. As I entered, Bob was conscious and confused. I got to spend a few moments with him, but then I met with the hospital's neurologist, Dr. John Mahoney, who could not have been kinder and more caring. He said he believed Bob had suffered a subarachnoid hemorrhage—a brain aneurysm. He said we needed to get Bob to a Boston hospital so he could have surgery, and he recommended Dr. Chris Ogilvy at Beth Israel. When Dr. Mahoney left the room, Sue and I googled Dr. Ogilvy, unsure if we should go to MGH or BI. We soon learned Dr. Ogilvy was one of the best of the best. So, with Dr. Mahoney's personal cell phone written on a piece of prescription pad paper in my pocket—just in case I had questions—I got into the ambulance with my husband for the ride to the hospital.

When we arrived at BI, they wheeled Bob into a room in the ER.

Sue and Rich were able to sit with me. We had sent the kids home, thinking that was the best place for them. Dr. Ogilvy came in a short while later. He confirmed Dr. Mahoney's diagnosis and said they would need to put a pump in Bob's head to drain the fluid building up in his head, creating dangerous pressure on his brain. He also needed to go in and repair the place where the aneurysm had burst. He drew a picture for me, depicting an aneurysm, and showed me how he intended to place a stent used in heart surgeries at the location of the aneurysm to allow the blood once again to flow through the blood vessel.

Okay, we have a plan.

By this point, Bob was now lying unconscious in his bed. We were waiting for an operating room to open up, but it was taking a while, and during that time, the pressure on his brain was building. We had waited a couple hours by this point, when Dr. Ogilvy and another doctor on his team came into the room and said we had to leave immediately. They said the pressure in Bob's head had become too much, and they could no longer wait for an OR. They were going to operate in the ER and put in the pump.

That's when I felt fear.

We went to a waiting room. I remember the procedure didn't take that long, and Dr. Ogilvy called to say it went fine and they would be bringing Bob to the OR to put in the stent. The stent procedure took longer, but thankfully, with the same result. Dr. Ogilvy came to the waiting room and said the operation went well; I could see Bob once they had settled him into the Neuro ICU. I gave Dr. Ogilvy a hug and then walked into an empty room, sank to my knees, and said a prayer of thanks.

Bob was not out of the woods. He would spend the next two weeks in the Neuro ICU in excruciating pain. The pump in his brain extracted a steady mixture of brain fluid and blood, reducing the pressure inside his skull. One night when his ICP (intracranial pressure) began to skyrocket, his main nurse, Kate—who was eight months pregnant at the time— called for a transport to bring Bob for a CT scan. The transport was taking a long time, and the pressure in Bob's head was at a dangerous level, so the very pregnant Kate hooked Bob up to mobile monitors and hauled his bed down to the CT room herself. *Amazing.*

I stayed by Bob's side most of the time but did take breaks when needed, especially as Bob would often times lash out at me. Yes, the man I loved
and was caring for; the man I was staying up all night with, listening for his
breathing and watching his monitors; the man I planned to spend the rest of
my life with would say horribly mean things to me for no apparent reason.

Fortunately, I had received two phone calls on the day of Bob's aneurysm that prepared me for this. My sister-in-law, whose husband had battled
terminal cancer, and a work friend, whose husband had had a stroke, both
warned me this would happen. It's not that he doesn't love you or that he is
angry with you," they said. "It's just he's hurt and in pain and can't lash out at
the doctors and nurses caring for him, so you end up bearing the brunt of it.

I am so grateful to have received that important heads-up, and I gladly
share it with others in similar situations. I also tell caretakers to carve out some
time each day, even if it's just a few minutes, to focus on you. I developed a
daily ritual. After the doctors came through on rounds, when I would listen to
their updates and ask my questions, I would then go outside and walk a block
to a coffee shop. There, I got myself a latte. I had never had one before, and I
don't know why I started ordering them then, but this ritual became my peace
in a world where I was scared but couldn't show it—a world where I needed
control but had none. In fact, for the first few months after Bob came home,
I would drive into town by myself on Sunday mornings, to that same coffee
shop near the hospital, to get myself a latte—it just made me feel better.

In the early days of Bob's Neuro ICU stay, the doctors told me they felt
he would pull through and make a full or nearly full recovery because he was
healthy to begin with. After a week or so, I started to believe that. Bob was getting better, and the pain inside his head was lessening. The nurses got him up
for walks, at first holding him up the entire time, but little by little, he started
to take steps on his own. After about twelve days, he was moved into a step-
down unit and prepared to come home.

Bob would need physical therapy and follow-up doctor appointments,
but he would be coming home.

The day we brought him home happened to be the final day of the annual members' tournament at the golf club to which Bob belonged. He had signed up to play before the aneurysm, and I know how disappointed he was to miss it—while being very happy to be alive. Bob loved golf and was a very good golfer, but we both knew he wouldn't be hitting the links anytime soon.

On the ride home, I decided to make a detour and bring him to the club. His sisters, who were there with us, thought I was crazy, but sometimes you just know what the best medicine is. He was weak and had to sit down the entire time, but he loved seeing all his golfing buddies and doing something normal again. Something that made him feel whole.

In the years since, my job has been to be the eyes and ears for Bob's head, as strange as that sounds. His doctor told me that he never relies on the patient to report how he's doing; he relies on the caregiver. You are the one to notice strange behavior, memory loss, or any other sign of trouble. So that is what I have done all these years—out of a sense of deep responsibility and much love.

SO HOW'S MY LITTLE GIRL DOIN'

by Lynda J. Tenaglia

Where do I begin this love story? I suppose I should start on the day I first laid eyes on you. Mike and I had been searching for the "perfect" puppy, visiting animal shelters every weekend. I wanted a puppy that was gentle, laid back, not too big, and easily trainable.

I was feeling a little "blue" on that fateful weekday in March 1991, so I decided to get out the yellow pages and just start calling shelters to see if any puppies were available. My second call hit the jackpot. They had a litter of seven puppies arrive that morning. Your mom was a purebred Beagle, and your dads were said to be German Shepherd and St. Bernard. What a combination!

We put the always-ready basket and blanket in the car and raced off to see if this would be the day. Well, there you were: the last of the litter left sleeping in the corner of the cage. You were so beautiful, all rolled into a tiny eight-week bundle of black-and-white fur. As I held you, your sleepy eyes began to open, and I asked you, "So how's my little girl doin'?" Once we put you down on the shelter floor, you became a blur of constant movement. You were so amazingly cute, and I immediately fell in love with your heart and soul. You were mine before I even filled out the paperwork. From that day forward, you were my little Jessica.

I must admit, I had no idea just how much work it was to raise and train a puppy. I dare say it was very similar to raising a child—a child that never grows out of the "terrible two-year-old" stage. But even when you were misbehaving, and in spite of all your mischievous ways, you were so adorable, intelligent, and fun.

Your energy saw no bounds, and we nicknamed you The Flying Wolanda early on. You would fly through the air at frightening heights with the greatest of ease. Sofa to the chair, back to sofa, and on and on until you collapsed in exhaustion. Heck, I was exhausted just watching you. And as if things weren't crazy enough, I had to deal with all your vocalizing. To this very day, I have no knowledge of any other dog that vocalized the way you did, Jess. I miss that so very much and would give anything to hear you talk back to me again.

The years ticked by, and my love for you grew. We made it through the usual illnesses and minor surgeries, and I was overprotective of you, just as I was with my children, Peter and Maria. There's no replacing the feeling of having children, but there is a special kind of unconditional love received from a dog. I had never known that kind of love in my life before you came along. No matter what I said, did, wore, or looked like, you loved me the same. We didn't fight or argue, though you did quite a bit of what I call grumbling. Not even my husband or children loved me the way you did.

You needed and wanted my constant attention, and I was happy to give it because you gave so much of it back to me. Whenever I sat down, you were there right next to me, so warm and cuddly. What a cuddle bug you were. I'd always ask you, "So how's my little girl doin'," and you would just cock your head and look at me with those sparkling brown eyes. That time together, especially after a long day at work, always recharged me so I could get dinner going and prepare for the evening ahead.

Now, let me talk about your kisses. Oh, your wonderful kisses. What a smooching fool you were. You had an attacking tongue that would seek out and lap at any part of the face. Not just your family's faces but our friends' faces as well. I witnessed unsuspecting victims try desperately to avoid your juicy darting tongue to no avail, only to have us all collapse in a fit of hysterical laughter. I think I miss your kisses the most, and the first thing I need when we meet again at The Rainbow Bridge is to hold you in my arms and feel your kisses smacking my face. I will keep that wish in my heart always, Jessie.

As the kids got older and left home for college and a life of their own, you and I spent more and more time together. Two "older girls" going through life side by side. I had many bleak days because of family issues, but you were always there to make me smile and feel safe. I am being honest when I say

I would never have made it through those days without you in my life. Every time I opened the door, you were right there jumping, wagging your tail wildly, and best of all, smiling as I asked, "So how's my little girl doin'?" Oh, that toothy grin of yours warmed my heart and made me laugh out loud no matter how tired or upset I may have been.

You made coming home so worth it. I can say that with all certainty because since you left this world, I find it very difficult to keep my head up during the bad days; coming home without you there to smile and greet me brings tears to my eyes. You brought a sense of peace and pure joy to my heart that I haven't been able to replicate in your absence. Who knew that my best friend would turn out to be you, my sweet Jessie? You were there through all the good and bad times for twelve years.

My years spent with you were special, but time started to take its toll on you. I watched as your muzzle turned gray, and your days of flying through the air from sofa to chair became less and less until they stopped. You stayed quite agile and spry, but I could see the subtle changes taking place, and it saddened me. I knew in my head that you couldn't stay with me forever, but my heart just wouldn't let me accept that you would ever leave.

At nine years old, your health started to decline a bit. You required more frequent visits to the vet and more gentle and attentive care at home to keep you feeling chipper. As it turned out, I left the job I had at the same time you were starting to feel your age, so I was home and able to spend more time with you. The extra time and care you needed was just fine with me.

Eighteen months before we lost you, sickness became a part of your everyday life. Infections seemed to overtake your little body. Vet visits and medications were a constant part of our lives, as well as cooking you a special bland diet. You were eating boiled hamburgers and rice so often now that I questioned the vet about the fact you were not getting the vitamins and nutrients needed to get better and stay healthy. We were assured you would be just fine, and sure enough, you would bounce back from each illness, only to get sick again in a couple of months. Soon, you were having fewer and fewer "good" days, and I began to panic inside. I never mentioned my fear to anyone at home. They knew I was very worried about all the problems you were having, but they were in denial. Actually, since I was the one taking care of you daily, it was easier for me to see the changes taking place. I desperately kept trying to make you healthy again, but it wasn't working.

When I went back to work, I found two part-time jobs. I worked 8:00 a.m. until noon at the first job, then rushed home, had a quick lunch, gave you a treat and a bathroom break, and then I was off to my second job. The months flew by, and life went on as usual. Dad and I took you with us on several weekend trips to Maine, New Hampshire, and Cape Cod.

After a few years of working two jobs, I wanted a change. Initially, I thought I wanted to become a cosmetologist. I enrolled at Elizabeth Grady School of Aesthetics, graduated, took the cosmetology exam in Boston, and received my license. But as it turned out, I accepted an offer for a job as an office manager for a home-based business. Stewart, my new employer, was a musician who played the Oboe and performed all over the country and sold musical-related articles to other musicians. The best part of the job was that it was very close to home, so I could be with you most of the time. The kids were finishing their college education, and our daughter, Maria, moved into her own apartment. I took you for more frequent walks and spoiled you with toys and homemade cookies.

During the Labor Day weekend in 2000, I was working on my computer with you right by my side. You seemed a little off that day, and when I looked down at you, I noticed that your mid-section looked swollen. I called the vet, who told me to bring you right in. We saw a new vet in the practice, and she gave us some medications to ease the pain, thinking you had a virus. Two days later, you were very sick, so I brought you back to the vet and saw Dr. Brian Borquin. Upon seeing you, he told me to rush you to the Woburn Animal Hospital because you had a very high fever.

After many tests, they told us you needed surgery to check for internal bleeding. They wanted to give us a cost estimate prior to the procedure, but we didn't care; we wanted our little girl to be healthy. They discovered you had hemangiosarcoma, which is cancer of the blood and blood vessels. We had a second opinion to see if chemotherapy would be an option, and the oncologist said that you could possibly live for another four months. Chemo-therapy wasn't a good option; it could give you more time, but there would be no quality in your life because of the side effects. Having you home was very sad and frightening. I watched you so carefully; I had no other priorities in my life. It was all about you every minute. I was so afraid of losing you.

The Christmas holidays were approaching, but my heart was not in it. We knew you were getting sicker, but you could still smile, kiss, and wag your tail for us. My heart was breaking; I asked you many times, "So how's my little girl doin'?"

New Year's Eve was very quiet. Dad and I stayed home that night to keep an eye on you. We felt the time was near when we would have to say good-bye. That night was long, and we never went to bed. We stayed in the family room with you stretched out on the sofa. The next morning was New Year's Day, and you had trouble standing and could not control your bowels. We wrapped you in a blanket and put you in the car. I sat in the back seat with you while we drove to Woburn Animal Hospital. We had a very kind veterinarian who explained the procedure of putting you to sleep. We didn't want to hear the news, but we knew it was your time, and to keep you would be selfish. It was so very heartbreaking.

While the doctor was preparing the room for us, you followed him around. You were looking for your pats on the head. He was very gentle with you. Walking into that room with you was frightening. I knew I would be without you forever. Dad, Maria, and I were with you while he carefully ad-ministered the needles—the last bit of pain you would ever feel.

When you were gone and finally at peace, the vet cut pieces of your fur for us to keep. We all kissed you and said goodbye. It was a very sad beginning to the new year.

Caregiving for Jess wasn't any different from caring for a parent, spouse, sibling, or child. The pain, exhaustion, fear, and sadness were the same; the amount of love and compassion we felt for her was the same; and the decision we had to make was the same as what humans face too—when does the pain and suffering of the treatment overshadow one's quality of life?

We never forget our loved ones, whether they be human or canine. They become part of our hearts and souls forever. Jessie left us more than twenty years ago, and I still think about her every day. During my darkest days, fighting my own cancer battle, I often turn to thoughts of her to help me cope. Just like I did all those years ago when she was by my side. Her kisses and brown eyes and wagging tale keep me going.

Since Jessie's passing, we adopted another little girl, Sophie. It was a rough beginning with Sophie, but in time, we became close, and she was my special friend throughout my battle with cancer. Sophie was an intuitive girl. She seemed to know there was something wrong with me even before my cancer diagnosis and found ways to show me that she cared. When I was not feeling well and lying down, Sophie would often lay by my side and place her head across my neck. I didn't know why, but her warmth felt good to me.

Several months later, after my ultrasound and visit with an oncologist, a tumor was discovered in the very spot where she lay her head. The tumor was malignant, and I would need radiation and chemotherapy treatments. After the tumor was removed and treatment began, Sophie never laid her head on my neck again, for she knew that it was being treated.

While undergoing treatment for cancer, I always found comfort and joy in Sophie, as I did with Jessie. Sophie lost her eyesight in the last four years of her life, but she always found a way to be beside me, to comfort me, especially when I was having a bad day. Throughout my many years of treatment, I have received love, comfort, and support from my family, as well as unselfish love and devotion from Jessie and Sophie—all of which have made my battles and struggles with cancer and treatments a little more bearable.

Lynda is a mother, grandmother and a ten year cancer survivor. Lynda is grateful to her husband, Mike, daughter Maria, son in law Aaron and grandchildren Abby and Jack for their caregiving and loving support. Also grateful for the ongoing care and terrific treatment received at Massachusetts General Hospital and Dana Farber Cancer Institute.

THE REALITY OF CANCER

by Alan E. Rubel

Like a million others before her, Sharon's cancer battle began with a routine checkup with her primary care physician. He noticed a small marking on her stomach, and even though she looked and felt great, he wanted to confirm it wasn't anything serious.

The scans shocked us all: her liver was loaded with tumors. Rather than immediately order a biopsy, her doctor encouraged us to get a second opinion. He was concerned that the biopsy might cause some bleeding, which could further complicate her condition.

The second doctor to see Sharon was at Brigham and Women's Hospital in Boston and his opinion differed completely. He thought that it looked more like blood tumors than cancer and he suggested we do nothing immediately, except monitor them monthly to see if there was progression, and determine which course of action to take. This was a relief in many ways, but we all knew what was lurking ahead.

During the beginning of Sharon's second year of scans, they did find something. She was sent to Dana Farber for additional testing. The results were more shocking than her primary diagnosis, especially in how they were delivered. Skipping the usual pleasantries, her doctor just blurted out, "You have liver cancer. I give you 3-6 months to live." We stared at one another in disbelief.

None of it made sense, and I pushed Sharon to seek a third opinion. Through a connection of our son, we got an appointment at Mass General Hospital. Three hospitals, three opinions. This time, the doctor had a little more tact in the delivery of his news.

"I have good news and bad news, but let's start with the bad ...you do have cancer. The good news is that it's not liver cancer. You have neuroendocrine cancer, which tends to be a slow-moving growth of the tumors. We'll do a scan once every other month and make decisions based on how fast the tumors are growing."

I was no expert in cancer types, but this one I had never heard of. According to the doctor, these tumors are cancers that begin in these specialized cells called neuroendocrine cells. Usually, this is a slow-moving cancer, but that doesn't mean much upon hearing the words *you have cancer*. We certainly had no idea what lay ahead, but Sharon, by nature, was extremely positive, and I would see that positivity play out hundreds of times over the next thirteen years.

Still, the reality of cancer had yet to sink in.

By Sharon's fourth scan, about eight months after her neuroendocrine cancer diagnosis, the tumors started growing. Instead of chemotherapy, however, her treatment involved receiving very painful shots. Sharon was supposed to get these shots every other month, but it quickly turned into every three weeks.

As Sharon's dosages increased over time, it became evident that a new course of action was needed. She began radioembolization treatment, which then required her to have radioactive beads inserted into her liver. Yes, radioactive, as in we couldn't sleep in the same bed or use the same bathroom for fear that I would be exposed! She was literally radioactive for a short time after these procedures, which happened three different times during her cancer battle.

A month or so after one of her procedures, we went to Montreal for the day. We had no trouble entering Canada but, on the way back in, the border patrol officer asked us what we were bringing with us into the United States.

"We have some food and small gifts, that's all."

"Are you bringing anything radioactive?" he asked.

"Absolutely not!"

"Well, the machines say otherwise. You're lighting up!"

It was a funny story to share after the fact, thinking these two old farts were sneaking radioactive material into the country, but not funny in real-time. It took a few hours for the doctors at Mass General and the border patrol to get on the same page.

The doctors were correct in one regard: it *was* a slow-moving cancer. Yet, five years into her treatment, Sharon's side effects worsened. She had severe chronic diarrhea and nausea, which caused major losses of potassium, low bicarbonate levels, and near-constant dehydration. Staying hydrated can be a challenge for healthy individuals, but if Sharon wasn't hydrated, she would literally die. As such, we were constantly in the hospital, either at Mass General or locally in Vermont, to put enough fluids into her body before she reached a point of no return. It was scary stuff, for me anyway, but Sharon never let it negatively impact her overall demeanor.

Don't get me wrong, Sharon could be a very stubborn woman—but that also saved her life. She had a burning desire to live. I would have done things differently at times, but as a caregiver, I needed to remember that it was *her* disease, not mine, and it was her decisions that guided us. Sharon had diabetes to contend with as well, which gave her peripheral neuropathy, causing painful pins and needles in her feet. There were times she would skip a set of medications and then try to convince me that she took them. I knew she hadn't, but again, it was her disease, not mine.

I always tried to be tender and gentle, but there were times I reached a breaking point and got testy, angry, or frustrated. Sharon would say something that would be very hurtful to me, but in time I realized that it was the cancer talking, not Sharon.

That's the reality of cancer.

We went to Boston every three to four weeks for thirteen years. It was 178 miles each way and the drive would take us four-to-five hours due to much-needed stops at rest areas. Most trips weren't easy. I would have a schedule for each travel day, but Sharon was on her own schedule. "Ten more minutes," she would often say, which turned into another hour! The trips themselves were beyond exhausting. and it got to a point where the car seemed to drive by itself, as the route became so familiar. It wasn't just the drive that became part of our routine. We got to know the parking garage, reception, and café attendants. We even got to know the panhandlers near the hospital. Dennis would greet us at the light, "Hi Sharon. Hi Alan."

The 50,000 miles we put on the car were the least of our problems. Because of her chronic nausea and vomiting, Sharon and I argued about the timing of her visits. There was no predictable schedule for them; some took place in the middle of the night and some during the middle of the day. "I want to see if I feel better before I get to the hospital." Or "I'm going to feel better." She never felt better. My take was, let me get you to the hospital so you *will* feel better. Her hydration visits were not five-minute fixes, either. I would pull up to the ER, go get the wheelchair, bring her in to check in, and then go park the car. It was a 3–5 hour treatment per visit, each time not knowing if they would let her go home.

There are different stages of cancer that the caregiver experiences. The first one is during the diagnosis. You're searching for as much information as you can get, and the questions far outweigh the answers. *Who do I call first? Do I get a second or third opinion? Is this really true?* It's a learning stage and one in which you develop your teams of doctors, family, and friends. Soon enough, you start realizing who's on and who's not on the team. Some people were unbelievably helpful. Others, not as much. It was hard to comprehend and accept that people have their own lives to live and we were not always top of mind. *Why aren't they making the phone calls and checking in more often?* It was very difficult to handle, and as much as we understood all of this, there were constant feelings of being alone in this fight.

The second stage is the planning one. How do you move forward based on the information available at that moment (especially as it constantly changes and evolves)? I became an "expert" in neuroendocrine cancer, embolization, diabetes, peripheral neuropathy and insurance nuances and policies. If we didn't have the right insurance, we could have lost everything. The cost of medication for a chronic illness is unbelievable.

Here's one example that still bothers me. Due to her chronic nausea, she took Zofran. One of the potential side effects of this drug was heart palpitations, which she began to experience. A cardiologist suggested we try a different drug called Emend.

"How come I never heard of this?" I asked him, as I knew every single medication that dealt with nausea.

"The reason is because it's a pre-chemo drug and Sharon never had chemo."

Sharon tried it in the hospital for the first time, and it worked well, but before she could start taking it full-time, the insurance company had to authorize it. Emend costs almost $3,000 a week—for four pills—and although I would have paid anything in that moment to give her a week of relief, at that cost, it would not have been sustainable. For six months I drove myself crazy trying to get her Emend; all the while, Sharon suffered greatly. After the insurance company finally approved her for the drug, I still had to figure out how to pay for it. It took countless hours of calls, emails and doctor assistance, but we got the cost down to $100 a week. It still bothers me today. We found a drug that kept Sharon out of the hospital and ER on a weekly basis, which cost pennies on the dollar compared to those hospital stays, and yet, I had to fight like hell to get the drug covered. Yes, the system is broken, my friends.

The drug did its job for three years, which was a big deal. Sharon still experienced nausea, but it wasn't chronic. By chronic, I mean getting up every couple of hours, having to experience diarrhea and vomiting at the same time. There was no such thing as a normal night's sleep. I slept with one eye open every night. Each time Sharon stirred, sat up, and headed to the bathroom, I wondered if it meant we were on our way to the hospital. Even if it wasn't to the hospital, I was up with her when she fought off the side effects and nausea. To this day, I still can't sleep through the night.

And the third stage many cancer caregivers go through is: Can we find a cure? I would talk to everyone. Anybody three steps away from me, I would talk about cancer, hoping someone would have some information for me. Sharon would get mad at me. She didn't want people to know what she was going through, but I didn't listen to her. I wanted to find a cure, find someone who had gone through this—I wanted so badly to find a cure. I should have honored Sharon's wishes to keep quiet about her cancer. I overstepped my boundaries and didn't listen to what she wanted. I'm not happy about it in hindsight, but I wanted her to beat this. I didn't want to lose her.

During the first five or six years of her battle with neuroendocrine cancer, Sharon and I had a beautiful life. We traveled, went out to dinner, and spent time with our fourteen grandkids. But the remaining years were brutal, especially her last two years. Those were long and hard days. No longer healthy enough to travel to and from Boston, she received treatment at our nearby hospital. She had good days, but it always led back to those violently ill episodes. Eventually, the chemicals and exhaustion wore her down.

That's the reality of cancer.

It was a thirteen-year battle for Sharon, and I'm still not sure how she stayed in the fight that long. I was emotionally and physically ruined by the end—but I wasn't the one with cancer. I did my best to support, advocate, listen, and love Sharon. I remember each time we arrived at Mass General, I put my best sales skills to the test and negotiated with her doctor to get her admitted to Lunder 9, the cancer floor. It was the equivalent of staying in a five-star Hotel. The nurses and staff were top-notch, knew Sharon well, and treated her like royalty. It was always worth the fight to get her there.

I also went out of my way to spend some time in the hospital chapel. It gave me some sense of hope. I remember one time asking God to show me a sign that Sharon will get better, then later saw a bumper sticker that read "Believe." It made me smile.

Sharon loved to shop. When she was feeling well enough to go shopping, I would drop her off at one of her favorite stores and wait for her in the car. "I'll only be 30 minutes," she said repeatedly, which turned into an hour or longer. She was always late. It used to drive me nuts, but it was her time to forget she had cancer and feel like a normal person.

My stress relief was throwing the javelin. It had been 60 years since I last threw the javelin, but it helped take my mind off the constant state of worry. I even entered myself into the Senior Games. When Sharon was in the hospital, I practiced. I got pleasure out of the physical challenge and competition.

One time, she went to a track meet with me, and it was very hot that day. I didn't want her to get heat exhaustion, so she watched from the car with the air conditioning on full blast. As it turned out, this was a longer than usual meet, and she ended up in the hospital the next week. I had so much guilt—about everything. It was hard not spending more time with our kids and grandkids. We would often have to miss holidays, birthdays, and games. The guilt that comes with caregiving is ubiquitous. It doesn't matter if the recipient of your care has cancer, dementia, or heart disease; the guilt is always there. It was for me, anyway.

Sharon's health could turn on a dime, and that was probably the hardest part of the entire journey. I never knew when her time would be called. One time the doctors told us she probably was not going to make it through the day, so Robert and I stayed overnight. The next morning, she was sitting up, reading the paper, impatiently waiting to be discharged. This happened more than once.

That's the reality of cancer.

Sharon's desire to fight and live was contagious. Each time she went into the hospital, she developed friendships with those around her. She encouraged them to keep fighting. It was just who she was, and she was very good at it. That's why you're reading this book.

While waiting for Sharon to go into recovery from one of her procedures, I was sitting and talking to Mike Tenaglia. I didn't know Mike until that day, but his wife Lynda was also about to go into recovery. The nurses called us in at the same time, and when we saw the women, they were already talking to each other. They became close friends, helping each other out with encouraging calls, texts, and emails. Mike and I became best friends as well and the subject of caregiving was something we always discussed. Sharing our experiences was helpful to both of us, and ultimately led to the creation of this book.

For the thirteen years of Sharon's treatments in Boston, we stayed with our son and his family. Although the trips were grueling, spending time either before or after the hospital with her grandkids, Lucy and Cole, were both the silver lining of a long journey and the best medicine. She received such tremendous joy in seeing them, and just as importantly, it gave her the opportunity to not think of herself as Sharon the cancer patient, but simply Grandma.

Our son Bobby and his wife, Jill played a huge role in caring for Sharon, and I would have been lost without them. No, more than lost—without the two of them, I would not have made it through Sharon's cancer battle. That's how big of a role they played. Not everyone is so lucky. It was an absolute gift to be with them and our grandchildren.

Unfortunately, they experienced a double dose of caregiving when Jill's mother was diagnosed with colon cancer in 2009. They hosted and cared for both of their mothers, many times at the same time—for eight years—before Ruth lost her battle in 2017. Bobby and Jill were our angels and Mitzvahs!

The month before Sharon died, in 2018, her doctor encouraged her to try a new type of shot.

"What else can I do?" she stated rhetorically.

The doctor had a response. He said, "I'm being direct with you: you don't have to take the shot. This is your choice. Only you can make the decision on your quality of life."

To Sharon—to all of us—the doctor's words gave her permission to die. She had always rallied after her trips to the hospital; she always had the burning desire to live. But this time, Sharon decided that she couldn't go on like this any longer. She had reached a point where she didn't have the strength to fight the cancer. The exhaustion and discomfort were too much. Whatever time she had left, she didn't want to use it on this uphill battle anymore.

I was torn by the doctor's statement. On the one hand, I was running on fumes. If Sharon was up at night, I was up with her. There's so much exhaustion and fear and uncertainty—every single day. It's dangerously unhealthy for the patient and caregiver.

I was so afraid of losing her and wasn't ready to admit defeat, but I knew I didn't have much left to give her either.

That's the reality of cancer.

The last day of Sharon's life was spent in a special room in the hospital, surrounded by the entire family. I was so exhausted. "Dad, go home. If anything happens, we'll call you. Get some rest."

I went home and fell asleep. In the middle of the night, there was a bolt of lightning inside me, and I sat up in bed. I looked at the clock. It was 3:07 a.m., and I knew that was when Sharon was going to die later that day.

The next day at the hospital, I just kept looking at the clock. 3:07 came and she was still alive. She died shortly after 5 pm. I don't know what the meaning of that bolt of lightning was, but I laughed at how Sharon even kept God waiting!!

The day after Sharon died, a woman came to my door; she woke me up actually.

"Is Sharon home?" she asked.

"I'm sorry to say she passed away yesterday," I replied.

This woman—a complete stranger to me—wept in my arms.

"I was in the bed next to her one time in the hospital. She was my motivation to get better—she told me to keep going, to keep fighting. I wouldn't be alive without her."

After Sharon passed, I began to realize what was important in life. We strive to be financially successful, but without your health and family, we have nothing. Now, I'm able to enjoy the beauty that surrounds me, something I failed to do before Sharon got sick. And all those little things that used to bug me incessantly in life—traffic, rude people, long lines, delayed flights, snowstorms...they don't bother me as much because they don't matter anymore.

Sharon was amazing. I'm not talking about her last visit to the hospital and how she made the decision to end her cancer battle with dignity and grace. I'm talking about the hundreds and hundreds of hours she spent in hospitals during her thirteen-year cancer fight. She spent more time motivating people, especially other patients, than she did worrying about her own condition. The battle she fought was inspirational to everyone around her.

As often as Sharon told me that I was her motivation to keep living, it was actually the other way around. She was *my* motivation. She inspired me every single day, long before she got sick and long after. Her sickness brought us closer. Our love grew deeper. We not only helped each other get through her cancer but also helped other people with their battles.

Being Sharon's caregiver was the hardest thing I have ever done in my life. Without hesitation, I would do it again tomorrow. The blessings of being her caregiver will never erase the pain and suffering I witnessed and often shared with Sharon, but there were many blessings for which I am grateful.

And that, too, is the reality of cancer.

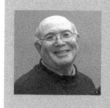

Alan E. Rubel is a Barre, Vermont resident and owner of Vision of Success, a Promotional Product & Printing company. A former board member of the Central Vermont Home Health & Hospice, Alan is also the Founding member of the VT Sports Hall of Fame, Publisher of *Vermont Gold*, and co-author of *Gloves* and *Love Letters to Sharon*. Alan is most proud of his 5 children, 14 grandchildren and 2 great-grandchildren.

"Life Isn't about surviving the storm but learning to dance in the rain."

THE LAW OF THREES

Anonymous

Whether it's a figure of speech or something more, we're all familiar with the notion of threes. I experienced mine over the course of three years.

At the age of seventy, I was fully employed and enjoying life as a musician, which allowed me to play several times a week. My world came to a crashing halt when I found my wife, Angie, on the bathroom floor at 4:00 a.m., her face collapsed. She had suffered a stroke.

After what we thought was a miraculous recovery, she soon started having seizures, and the grueling process of finding the right seizure medication began. During this time, she was scared to death of being home alone, so I left my music behind and cut back my work schedule to be with her. Her three-year battle with seizures and grueling side effects from the medication prompted many trips to the ER. During one of those visits, a chest X-ray suggested that she might have lung cancer. She did.

Angie's three-year "trip" taught me a lot. I learned that being with Angie through the sickness and death was a peak experience—even better than music. I learned the value of staying positive. Angie and I never gave up on an eventual recovery until just two days before she passed away. I learned more about love during her sickness than our prior forty-two years of marriage had taught us.

Caregiving is just that—it's love; it's natural. I wouldn't trade my caregiving experience with Angie for anything in the world.

* * *

Our son Matt was an alcoholic and a very tough patient.

Alcoholism progressed over the course of his life to the point where there was very little positive between us. We had terrible fights, sometimes physical, and my thoughts toward him bent all the rules of love. I often saw him as a lost soul and was packed with resentment.

Through all this turmoil, my love—however nebulous—continued. I prayed for his sobriety, mustering positive thoughts of what he had once been and could become. I paid for multiple rehabs—yes, I know enabling is taboo, but it's always done in the name of love—but in Matt's case, it wasn't meant to be. At the age of forty-one, he went out in the woods, numbed himself with alcohol, laid down, and died of exposure.

This case may hardly seem like caregiving, but I would argue that it was the only style of caregiving Matt's illness would allow. I did what I could for Matt, and yes, love plus caregiving were indeed key ingredients.

* * *

My dog Maggie died of old age. She was fourteen, and it was the most natural death of the three.

Maggie, a gentle soul, became my soulmate after Angie and Matt died. During my time of grief, I constantly asked myself, "Why Angie? Why Matt?" I would turn to Maggie and ask "Where's Angie? Where's Matt?"

We helped each other. We bonded. As her hips became lame and her panting spoke of increased pain, my third caregiving experience began for me. I found a gentle vet who made multiple home visits. There were pills, expensive pills, bone-strengthening chewies, and special senior food. I even brought in a baby crib mattress to replace her worn rug.

Maggie's dotage lasted a whole year until one morning when her hips refused to let her rise. I called that same gentle vet, and Maggie was allowed to finally sleep in peace.

* * *

That's my tale—a tale that focuses on death but contains overwhelming love. Death's multiple personalities expose agony, frailty, and sometimes tragedy—but I'm a believer. I believe souls go on to wonderful places, and no one's sure how that works.

I also believe that caregiving has made all the difference in my life.

THE DEATH OF ME

by Craig Martin

For the love of mom and all other things holy.

My mother has a beauty that never fades

Her face, for all her years, is untouched by age

Her face reflects her kindness, her dignity, her grace

Time has been less lenient with my mother's mind

I've watched her memory fade, and I've watched her thoughts slide

As I've learned to listen, to hear, to properly attend

I've seen what a mind rooted in reality cannot comprehend

What happened yesterday is jumbled with days gone by

A lifetime of years happening all at once through my mother's eyes

One day my mother and I were children together

Playmates, best friends

Perhaps my mother has seen the hereafter, the end

Her own father is back with us at times

Giving comfort, advice, and the occasional corny line

The line of her thoughts does not run straight

The garden of her memories opens through multiple gates

The connections run from lessons learned

To things and people loved, places and times for which a young girl's heart still yearns

I'm not sad to see a lifetime through this muddled lens

I'm grateful I've learned to properly attend

It was my normal Thursday night dinner with mom.

It would still be a few years before the things we noticed would be called Alzheimer's. Right now, the purses left behind at restaurants, the moments of disorientation, the names that couldn't be matched to faces were just "something's up with mom." Thursday was my stepfather Jim's bowling night, and while so far, nothing bad had happened with mom, we both decided she shouldn't be left alone. Jim was willing to give up his bowling night, but I wanted him to keep his sanity. I also saw an opportunity to spend regular, quality time with my mom while I still could and while she could still appreciate it.

After the appetizer plates were cleared and we sat waiting for the main course, Mom's eyes drifted over to the bar where a group of young men was congratulating each other heartily on some success of the day. Her gaze disappeared somewhere far away, and I could see her struggling to remember something just at the edge of consciousness. Something was right there, but somehow, it was also just out of reach. She looked down at the table, trying to find what eluded her mind.

She shrugged her shoulders after a bit and sighed deeply. "For years, I thought my youngest would be the death of me," she began. It was clear she wasn't aware of who her audience was, but I let her continue the story because by now, I've already learned that correcting her upsets her, and also because, as her youngest, I was rather curious to see where this story about her youngest would go.

"I swear to God, I worried myself sick about that kid. He just could never sit still. I couldn't take my eyes off him for even a second. The minute I did, he was out swimming over his head, jumping off rocks, disappearing into the woods, and running off God knows where. I loved him to death, but I also thought he was going to give me a heart attack. And the worst part was knowing that if I died of a heart attack, I wouldn't be there to save him from his damn self anymore. Good Lord, thank God we got through that, because seriously, I thought he would be the death of me."

I had a wry smile counterbalanced with moist eyes as I quietly listened to this accurate description of my younger self. Slowly, Mom looked up from the table and fixed her eyes on mine. Gradually, a look of comprehension came over her face, and she broke into a wide grin, letting out one of her loud, signature laughs that everyone in the restaurant heard and many in the restaurant recognized from our other Thursday night dinner dates. "Oh, for Christ's sake!" she exclaimed. "It was you!"

That was five years ago. There are no more dinners out. Mom only leaves the house for short walks around her condominium complex. Thursday nights, I sleep over on the pullout couch I got for her bedroom; restaurant dinners belonged to a time now passed. Her bedroom used to be the living room, but the living room is the only room that doesn't require her to go up and down stairs, so now the living room is her bedroom. It's next to the kitchen, and these two ground-floor rooms constitute virtually her entire universe.

Where she once had a collection of cosmetics many women would kill for, she now has a bin full of adult diapers. Her childhood doll collection sits in the corner of the room in a baby buggy she sometimes pushes around that small, two-room universe. Once in a while, she still tells me stories. More often, she tells the stories to her dolls. Occasionally, I still hear her loud, signature laugh, but these days, it's her who is going to give me a heart attack.

It's cliché to say our roles are reversed, but that's what's happened. Mom's story in the restaurant wasn't wrong—I wasn't an easy kid, and I was worse as an adolescent. I definitely did all the things she talked about and a lot of things she never found out about. On a college campus tour at eighteen, I actually ran away from the tour group because I was more interested in exploring the woods adjacent to campus than being shown the library. When I eventually attended that college, I spent more time between the trees than I did between the stacks.

Thirty-four years later, I still remember the resigned look on my mother's face when I eventually rejoined the tour group as if nothing was out of the ordinary. Despite all that, this woman who now needs my help to go to the bathroom, who we've removed the knobs on the stove for, whose teeth I have to brush, loved me ferociously and without reservation.

My mother thought I would be the death of her, but she also thought nothing of the possibility of dying for me. Over time, as I've lost the mom that I thought I knew, I've found the one I should have known all along. At long last, I can see the mom who suffered silently as I broke her heart over and over. At long last, I can see the mom who continued to love me ferociously and without reservation through all that heartbreak, even when she thought it would kill her. I see all this because I've learned that I'm capable of the same.

I gained some appreciation for what my mom did for me when I had kids of my own, but I didn't appreciate all she did until I had to do it for her. It isn't just about taking care of her daily physical needs; it's about being her emotional protector. Alzheimer's has turned her world into a scary place. Of all the things I do for my mom during this time of difficulty, the greatest of them is telling her how much I love her and promising her that she will always be safe, even as she occasionally puts herself in danger.

About a year before COVID-19 reached the US, Jim and I had bought a three-generation house to help take care of Mom together. The layout of the house was perfect for what we needed. The first floor had a suite for Mom and Jim with a large bedroom and full bathroom. Upstairs had three bedrooms and another full bath. We shared the kitchen and living room. For some time, the arrangement worked very well, but eventually, it became too much for all of us.

My dogs have an energy level that isn't compatible with Alzheimer's. Having three generations all feeling like the walls were closing in during the isolation of the pandemic wasn't working either. First, Mom and Jim went back to their condo down the street, and then we made the decision to move Mom to an assisted living facility. We had done our best for Mom's sake, but eventually, both Jim and I were pouring from empty pitchers. It was time. Transferring mom to an assisted living facility seemed like the right thing to do.

The folks at the facility assured us that they were experts in memory care and capable of taking care of mom. They didn't love her, though. They couldn't promise her that her feelings were safe. She wasn't their Mom.

When Mom felt scared and needed help, they gave her increasingly powerful sedatives and put a note in her file saying she was difficult. Eventually, they sent my mother to a psychiatric emergency room without so much as calling me. Psychiatric emergency rooms are no fun under the best of circumstances. In the height of the COVID-19 pandemic, it was a nightmare.

When I learned what happened and raced to the hospital, there was little I could do. I sat by my mother's side for two days, poorly singing Joni Mitchell's *Both Sides Now* to keep Mom calm while all around her, people in various states of emotional crisis, including inmates from the nearby county prison, screamed and yelled and threatened the staff.

I risked arrest by refusing to move from the foot of my mother's bed when the shift coordinator wanted to transfer Mom upstairs to their extended stay ward—where visitors weren't allowed. Fortunately, the MPs on loan from the Air Force base to provide hospital security had watched me sing to my mom, cry by her side, and simply be there with her. By the time they were asked to handcuff me and take me away from my mother, they had made up their minds to slowly step out of the room and pretend they didn't hear.

When I was finally able to speak to the physician in charge and convinced him to release Mom into my care, I put her in a wheelchair and sprinted to the exit before anyone could change their mind. I drove straight past the assisted living facility, and I brought my mom home where she would be loved.

On that day, I thought my mother would be the death of me. I also thought nothing of dying for her.

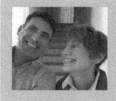

Craig Martin has been a businessman, a father and a philanthropist. Now he spends most of his time as a caregiver to his mom while writing stories, poems and essays when possible. Everything he has been and is he owes to his mother.

ONE SMALL DOSE

by Deb Kimberg

Caring for my son with autism spectrum disorder has morphed numerous times over my son's eighteen years. We had no idea what was in store for us.

As a young child, my son was a twohead, happy, and high-energy child. At preschool, he enjoyed playing with friends in the classroom and on the playground, and especially charming his teachers. He was known as a class clown and well-liked.

However, there were always signs that something was just not quite right. When he was tired or bored, he had an unusual movement in which he moved his chin to his chest and slowly rolled his head back to the left-hand side—over and over again. Additionally, coordination was difficult for him, and he showed no interest in sports. Even something as simple as playing on the playground presented a challenge. He refused to climb up playground equipment with steep open stairs unless an adult braced his core until he got to the top, then insisted someone hold his hand to cross the bridge.

We didn't worry too much about these oddities. He seemed to be doing well enough. Sadly, as he continued to age, his differences from the other children became more glaring.

In elementary school, he struggled. He was hyper, silly, and unfocused, which made concentrating on schoolwork a challenge. He was quickly placed in special education for a slew of special education services including reading, occupational therapy, and social skills. In these early years, he developed some other odd behaviors, such as hand flapping when he was happy and frequently using silly, babyish words when he spoke.

An ADHD diagnosis promptly followed along with medication to treat it, which made him a shell of himself. My happy, silly son became quiet and sullen. Furthermore, the medication suppressed his appetite, so we had to time meals between doses so he could get the nourishment he needed. After beginning the medication, it became difficult for him to gain weight. Although he was calmer, with the restrictions in mood and behavior, making friends became more difficult.

It soon became clear that my son was a special needs child who was on the autism spectrum.

Caring for a child on the spectrum was demanding on our family and work lives. It also required that we be heavily involved at school to ensure my son received proper accommodations, seeking private tutoring and therapies, and helping to facilitate play dates to encourage friendships.

Still, we enjoyed many fun times with our family. We spent evenings and weekends shuttling his two older brothers to their soccer practices and games, then enjoying burgers and shakes at Sonic afterwards. Although not perfect, life was normal enough, and we all enjoyed our family time.

Unfortunately, as a young teen, my son's behavior began to worsen. The changes came on insidiously over the course of a year. He became a recluse in his room, playing video games and watching YouTube incessantly, only to come out to attend school or eat a meal. My previously sweet child often was angry, rude, and demanding. Then, he began to grunt, squeal, and stammer. With his learning challenges, he was falling further behind in school each year. And with his baby talk and immature behavior, his social skills were similarly falling more behind each year.

We didn't know what adult life would be like for him—or for us.

Then, during winter break one year, I read the book *Brain on Fire: My Month of Madness* by Susannah Cahalin. I was amazed that this young woman developed an infection in her brain that caused her to develop a slew of debilitating psychiatric and physical symptoms over the course of one month. Her case was a medical mystery. As a last-ditch effort, a neurologist was brought in from University of Pennsylvania, who tested her for a rare condition called anti-NMDA receptor encephalitis, which, luckily for her, was positive and led to proper treatment and recovery.

Intrigued by Cahalin's story, I sought out an appointment with an integrative medical doctor. At my son's initial appointment, the doctor indicated that she suspected that my son also had a type of autoimmune encephalitis that was contributing to his symptoms associated with autism. Testing showed that he likely had multiple infections associated with Lyme disease, and most importantly, a little-known infection called Bartonella, sometimes referred to as Pediatric Acute Neuropsychiatric Disorder (PANS). Though, his symptoms were not acute. After reviewing the long list of potential symptoms, surprisingly, I realized I had mild symptoms throughout my life, too, and likely transmitted these stealth infections to him during pregnancy.

At the time and even today, seven years later, this is a hotly debated diagnosis. Nonetheless, I was encouraged that we had a new avenue to pursue, rather than just accept the commonly held notion that "my child was just born this way." With a diagnosis to embrace and treat, caregiving for my son turned a corner again to include helping him heal from these little-known infections with insufficient research on effective treatment.

My son tried multiple antibiotic treatments, many of which made his behavior worse and were quickly abandoned. *How could antibiotics make my son's symptoms worse?* The doctor assured us this happens sometimes and is a good sign that the infections were dying off and causing his behavior to temporarily flare.

My family was skeptical, especially since none of our other doctors agreed with the diagnosis or knew anything about it for that matter.

As my son's behavior continued to worsen, symptoms increased to include OCD, oppositional behavior, obsessiveness, and multiple occurrences of trying to run away. My husband and I were at our wits end.

Despite many failed treatments, I became a fierce, determined momma. My caregiving transformed from focusing on therapies to help my son manage his autism symptoms in school and at home to finding a medical treatment to help him feel better, though I didn't know what that could mean for him.

After five years of little progress, we had given up all hope for any type of improvement in him. After years of failures and exhausting the treatment options doctors had recommended, I began working to get him on disability after high school and searching for any kind of work he could do as an adult with special needs.

And then, in a shockingly sudden development, our persistence paid off.

An existing drug was identified by Dr. Jayakumar Rajadas at Stanford that changed my son's life. After one small dose, the worst of his behavior had a swift and remarkable improvement. He became happier and more social, coming out of his room often to hang out with the family. His safety was no longer a concern as he stopped threatening to run away.

Before long, his picky eating disappeared, and he began eating everything. This slight sixteen-year-old gained thirty pounds over six months. He transformed physically from an anemic-looking child who could blow away in the wind to a healthy, thriving teenager.

With another set of antibiotics that he couldn't tolerate earlier, he suddenly experienced a resolution of eight tics, including grunting, squealing, stammering, and throat clearing, and his hyperactivity dissipated.

Soon after, we noticed something even more surprising. Nine months into treatment, his learning disabilities and attention deficit were resolved. In less than a year, his reading comprehension moved from a fifth-grade level to on track for tenth-grade on state-wide testing. And in a completely unprecedented occurrence, my son and my son's high school teachers came to the realization that he no longer needed the support of special education. Consequently, the school removed his special education support at the beginning of eleventh grade. It was a tearful moment for everyone who supported him at school.

Also striking was that his baby talk and age regression resolved. Not only did he look like a thriving high school student, but he was also interested in making friends, getting his driver's license, and going to college. This was unthinkable one year earlier.

With so many improvements, my focus as a caregiver morphed again into something that had no roadmap. Now that my son was suddenly performing at grade level and wanted to attend college, my energy turned to helping him catch up on many lost years of learning. Our family was blessed to find an ACT tutor who fell in love with my son's story and was up for the challenge, one of the biggest of her long career.

Against all odds, by a stroke of luck and our family's fierce determination, my son was accepted into a four-year college.

It was a long, difficult, and expensive journey that took seven years, ten doctors and practitioners, countless failures, and tens of thousands of dollars.

To be clear, my son remains on the autism spectrum, mostly due to social awkwardness and shyness. We expect that he'll always be somewhat on the spectrum and will need some support.

So, next year, my caregiving will change again. What support will my son need to be successful with schoolwork and living independently in college? Our current plan is to keep him on long-term antibiotic treatment until doctors can find a way to clear the infections. When we've tried pulling him off his medicines in the past, his symptoms return within days. Will he remember to take his medication daily so he can continue to function at a high level?

My job as a caregiver may never end—and that's okay.

Despite no help from our standard medical care team consisting of our pediatrician and neurologist, I know that I did everything I could to help my son lead his best life. And I pray that science catches up to help many other children suffering with unsuspecting stealth infections leading to their symptoms associated with autism.

Debbie Kimberg, living in Dallas, TX, is a busy mother of three boys and an executive in the financial service industry. She has spent the past seven years helping her children and herself recover from ASD, ADHD, and other psychiatric issues caused by stealth infections that were overlooked by traditional medicine. She also works with multiple Lyme foundations and is an administrator of multiple Facebook groups on Tick-borne Disease, PANS, and autism. You can follow her son, Sammy's journey on Instagram, TikTok, and FB at @HijackedBrains.

LOSING YOUR BEST FRIEND TO CANCER

by Sara Robinson

with Mark J. Resnick

My parents started smoking as teenagers, like many in their generation did. I was never on an airplane when smoking was allowed, but there always seemed to be a cloud of smoke hovering above us in our Brighton duplex. I never thought much about it, even when I was a teenager myself.

I had stepsiblings from my dad's first marriage but was an only child for my parents. There was no doubt that I was daddy's little girl. Despite him owning two businesses and working long hours, we were a very tight-knit family. But when my dad died suddenly in 2000, Mom and I became even closer.

There was nothing wrong with my dad when he died, and there was nothing he could have done to prevent his death. It was a stomach aneurysm that killed him. By the time I left work and got to the hospital, he was dead within the hour.

Although smoking had nothing to do with my dad's passing, Mom quit smoking immediately. Cold turkey. I'm guessing she did it for me—or, more specifically, so I wouldn't have to worry about losing another parent prematurely due to her smoking habit. She always had the best intentions.

After college, I continued to live with my mom. Of course, we lived our own lives, but she was very much a part of my life and vice versa. There wasn't much we didn't know about each other. From a health perspective, Mom was healthy. The only issue she had was a cyst on her kidney, which was monitored each year by her doctor.

In the summer of 2014, Mom had her annual scan for the cyst on her kidney, only this time, the doctor found something. The kidney was fine, but there was a spot on her lungs. A few days later, via a telephone call, she heard the three words you never want to hear: *You have cancer.* It was stage 3 lung cancer, but because she was alone when the call came in, Mom started to freak out. She called a close friend who, fortunately, calmed her down.

Like the sudden passing of my dad, this was shocking news for Mom and me. She wasn't the slightest bit sick or off her game in any way. She owned a successful antique store in Allston and loved her customers. She was happy. In fact, we spent most of the month talking about my cousin's upcoming wedding in Nantucket.

Within a matter of days, Mom settled down and then took charge. She immediately put the house and other accounts in my name so I wouldn't be burdened by these issues if she got really sick. Once that initial shock wore off, she became very positive. She kept her happy persona and near-constant smile on her face. And as expected, she didn't tell anyone about her diagnosis because she didn't want them to feel sorry for her, including John and everyone at the wedding.

After John's wedding, Mom had surgery to remove the cancer. It was close to the aorta, but they were able to get it out. That was great news, and we both felt more optimistic about the prognosis. It was only after the surgery that a new doctor corrected her stage—it was stage 4, not 3 like she was initially told. Still, she remained positive.

Mom did chemotherapy for six weeks, but it was the first dose that sucked the most. She was constipated, agitated, exhausted, and in pain. It took a couple of days to recover each time she had the chemo. After her third treatment, I asked her doctor for another type of chemo, one that didn't constipate her so much. That was an important lesson to learn—if you don't ask questions—or question the treatment options—your loved one might suffer unnecessarily.

Radiation was next. This was difficult for my mom because you need to stay very still during the treatment. That lasted six weeks, but she would do radiation any day over chemotherapy.

Upon completion of both treatments, we received good news: the cancer was in remission, meaning it hadn't gotten larger or spread to other part of her body. Mom was excited, like she had gotten her life back. If anything, it bought her more time.

We returned to Beth Israel Hospital every three months for checkups. What an awful feeling it was each time we entered the hospital for those appointments. You can't help but think the worst, no matter how positive one is. And for a year and a half, all was good. It wasn't until her seventh follow-up appointment that she got the next set of words you never want to hear: *The cancer is back*.

There were no obvious signs of the cancer's return until many months later. One morning, Mom couldn't get out of bed. She couldn't walk. I called the ambulance and took her to the hospital, where she remained for three days. Each night, the nurses would ask her a series of questions, and sometimes she had trouble answering them. My mom called me at work the next day and said, "They think the cancer went to my brain, and you know what that means."

"Why do they think it went to your brain?" I asked.

"Because I had trouble with some of the answers last night when they woke me up."

You have to be kidding me? I was very unhappy with her medical team for saying that to my mom. They ran more tests, and they came back fine. Her white blood cell count was still down, so they did a spinal tap. Nothing.

Finally, I asked the nurses, "Is it possible her white blood counts are down because she hasn't eaten or had anything to drink the past eight hours due to all this testing?" When they gave her juice and crackers, her counts came back up. But she wasn't out of the woods yet.

The follow-up scans they did on this visit showed that the cancer had spread. Not to her brain but to her legs. It wasn't a large mass, so she would only have to undergo radiation, not chemo.

Three radiation treatments helped contain the spread—for a while.

At her three-month follow-up, they found a blood clot in her leg. When we left the hospital, I had a package of needles and a bucket for the used syringes so I could give her shots to break up the clot.

"You want me to give her the shots? I can't do this; I'm a teacher, not a nurse."

But they walked me through it, and I gave Mom her first shot in the stomach before leaving that day. I then gave her a shot every morning on the right side of her stomach; at night, I gave her a shot on her left side. *It was terrifying.* I felt like I was hurting her, but she said I wasn't.

Two weeks of shots to her stomach cleared up the blood clot, which was a good thing, as her entire stomach was black and blue, and I had run out of clean space to give her any more shots.

During her remaining treatment, Mom didn't ask much about her prognosis. She didn't want to know. There were good days and bad. On a return trip to the hospital to treat another bout of severe constipation, they told us the spots on her lungs had gotten larger and she would need more chemo. That's when she said to me, "I don't want to do this right now. I want to take a break." I think she knew all along that her body wasn't right.

When the doctor asked to speak to me alone, I was surprised. I had no idea why she wanted to see me. I went to the waiting room, and she told me it was time to consider hospice for my mom.

"What? Hospice. Why?"

"It's time," she said.

"But we just came in for constipation."

"The cancer has spread. It's all over her body now."

"How long does she have?"

"Two weeks to two months."

I broke down right in front of the doctor. Then I asked her not to tell my mom. I didn't want her to know that she was dying; I didn't want her waking up each morning wondering if this was the day she would die. The doctor's next statement surprised me all the same.

"I've never met such a brave young woman like you who has stepped up like this."

I didn't feel brave or young, and she wasn't just my mom—she was my best friend.

My next call was to work. I told them I wouldn't be coming in until my mom died. Then I called my Uncle Barry, Mom's only sibling, and gave him the news. A few more phone calls and I was back in the room.

"What's up?" she asked.

"Nothing, just some paperwork stuff. Nothing to worry about."

But she knew.

"I want you to know something," she said. "I want you to know that your cousins will be there for you no matter what."

For the third time that morning, I was surprised. I didn't have a close relationship with my cousins, all three of whom were many years older than me. I only really saw them at holidays.

"We're not even close, Mom. I can't just pick up the phone and call them."

"Believe me, Sara. They will be there for you."

"Okay, Mom. Thank you," I replied with an eye-roll to keep things light.

Mom left the hospital with a walker. When we got home, she went straight into the living room and into her favorite chair. I didn't know which hospice group to call, so the hospital made those arrangements. I asked them not to tell my mom that this was the end; that she was dying.

"If she is of sound mind, I need to ask her certain questions," the woman from hospice said.

"No—you don't. I am telling you what she wants," I pleaded with her.

This particular hospice worker was very direct and rude to Mom. After what seemed like a minute of questioning, Mom blurted, "Get the fuck out of my house!"

My friend Scott gave us the number of a new hospice group, and they were helpful and very nice. They gave Mom sponge baths and asked about a hospital bed instead of sleeping on the recliner.

"Do you want them to bring in a hospital bed?" I asked Mom.

She replied, "Do you want a hospital bed, Sara?"

"No."

"Then why the fuck do I want one."

As I've heard from many other caregivers of loved ones with cancer, it's not always the person who is talking—*It's the cancer*. And it was.

"Sara, am I sick?"

"Yes."

"Really sick?"

"Yes, Mom."

"I'm going to fight it!"

Right up to the end, she still had her sense of humor. The next day her brother, Barry, came to visit. Mom had an accident just prior to his arrival and started crying.

"I don't want him to see me like this!" she sobbed.

"It's fine, Mom. We'll get you cleaned up, and he'll never know."

Days later, Mom said to a friend, "I'm tired. I can't do this anymore. I'm just tired."

Hospice said it could be forty-eight hours, so I called some people so they could come by and say goodbye. The next day, Mom was looking up at the ceiling and called me over.

"I love you, Sara."

"I love you too, Mom."

Within minutes after our exchange, she went into a coma.

I asked everyone to leave so I could have some alone time with her. I appreciated the wisdom of the hospice nurse who told me that "the hearing is the last thing to go, so talk to her."

If you've done this before for loved ones, then the words will be all too familiar, though just as hard to read, I'm sure.

"You gave it a good fight, Mom. It sucks you lost it, but you fought hard. And you're right, my cousins will be there for me. I love you so much and am proud of you."

She squeezed my hand every so slightly—at least, I think she did.

"It's time for you to go."

I went to bed that night on the couch. At 11:00 p.m., she was still breathing. At 1:00 a.m. in the morning, something woke me up. I checked on Mom, and she wasn't breathing any more. She was gone. I turned the oxygen off and sat with my mom.

The hardest part of my caregiving experience was not being able to help her with the pain and watching her suffer. I also felt bad that she couldn't enjoy life anymore. Funny enough, we still fought during her illness, but we never stopped being best friends.

I lost my mom but got my cousins back. I am now very close to them. They were there for me every step of the way, just as Mom promised. It's when tragedy strikes that you see who your real friends and family are— and who stays with you after the event. I'm not sure I could have coped with Mom's death without my cousins.

My mom died in 2017. I still live in the same house. The clouds of smoke are long gone inside the home, but outside, I often see Mom's smile in the clouds high above. Or I'll feel her presence while watching TV in the living room in which she passed.

Sometimes, when I get off the phone with one of my cousins, I find myself turning in the direction of where her recliner used to be to say, "You were right, Mom."

LET ME HUG YOU

by Ana Peach

I remember listening to Joan Lunden talk about caretaking for an elderly parent, and I must say, that even as sensitive as I was about the issue, it was foreign to me. I was probably in my mid-forties at the time. Then my dad died, and I became the sole caretaker for my mother, who was seventy-eight years old.

Everything Ms. Lunden had described more than twenty years ago—the joy and stress, the burdens and blessings, and the overwhelming range of emotions experienced each day—was suddenly my reality.

While caring for my mom, she went from being an independent, determined, strong-headed, fun-loving widow to a person who, other than appearances, I would not recognize. Dementia robbed me of the last six years of enjoying my mom as I had always known her. She became the child, and I became the parent. She went from being the person in charge to the one who had to be prompted when to eat, walk, and get tucked into bed at night.

Yet, as my mother's dementia progressed, she developed dysphagia and was unable to eat solids, except bananas and Madeleine cookies, which were very soft and would melt in her mouth. For the past seven years, I puréed her meals, not only so she could eat but also so that I could accurately track her calorie intake to maintain a healthy weight. Offering her tasty meals became a challenge, but I was lucky she didn't mind the soups and meals in liquid form.

During this stage of dementia, I kept a baby monitor and an alarm clock on my nightstand. The monitor was a godsend, but there were many nights I thought I heard her talk, move, or walk around the floor. I spent most of the night awake to see if I needed to run downstairs and take care of her needs, which I did every night.

137

My mother never wet her Depends. Instead, she would take them off before heading to the bathroom, only to urinate on the way there, unable to control her bladder. I was told it had to do with dignity. Every night, I mopped the floor between the bedroom and bathroom until I started tracking her sleep patterns. I set my alarm for two and a half hours after she went to bed so that I could take her to the bathroom. Then, two and a half hours after that, I repeated the process until morning time. Three to four times a night, I woke up to get her to the bathroom.

I felt guilty waking her from a sound sleep, then carrying her to the toilet. But I also needed to keep her on a schedule to help stop the accidents and from washing floors in the middle of the night. It was tough on my emotions and my physical being, no doubt. Often, I would fantasize with the idea of placing her in a facility, but I always resolved to keep her at home until a future date, when I knew I couldn't possibly do it any longer.

Yet despite relying on me for her care, Mom was able to run away from our home to nearby houses, go up and down several staircases dozens and dozens of times each day, and dance up a storm when people were gathered in celebration. My mother was full of action and sharpness, a woman full of confidence who made everyone feel liked and appreciated.

She never thought, *What will they think about me?* And she was so genuinely herself, one hundred percent of the time. I used to say to myself sometimes, "ignorance *is* bliss!" She lived her life the way she wanted to, and she even passed away while doing something that she liked very much—sweeping and preparing the surroundings for a family gathering.

My mother's existence in the last few years was amazing. I would arrive home, and she would ask, "Now, who are you?" I told her my name and who I was, to which she replied, "My Ana Maria?" I nodded, and she became so happy, then said, "Let me hug you!"

When that minimal interaction ended about six months prior to her final days, I became obsessed with trying to bring back some of her memories. I constantly talked to her, even though I knew she couldn't understand and knowing I wouldn't get any answers back. I was blessed because I learned so much from her about myself, my family, life, and existence. And she was blessed because she could not have been loved any more; she could not have been better taken care of by her family. My mom showed us all how to belong in the midst of every generation, social status, or educational level.

I hurt a great deal from her loss, but I remind myself that she lived one hundred years, five months, and twenty-two days. But who is counting? I have almost seventy years of memories of a great woman. When I feel frustrated about this terrible disease that robs so many of great moments and memories with their elderly parents, I am grateful for opportunities like this to share her with the world—to celebrate her.

WHY I NEVER HANG UP THE PHONE ANGRY

by Julie Doherty

with Mark J. Resnick

It was a Sunday morning. In the early afternoon, we were leaving for a week-long vacation to Cape Cod. My husband Phil and I fought over his decision to check on a job site before leaving for the Cape. His crew was working seven days a week on this project, and he wanted to check in with the crew one more time. He called me from the job site, and I was annoyed that he was still there. We argued, and I hung up the phone angry—no, I was furious. What was so important that needed his personal attention? The company knew it was his vacation week—only it wasn't them who insisted he stop at the site; it was Phil. That's just how he was wired.

Mid-morning on April 15, 2018, I got the call. Phil was in an accident at work. I was told he got hit by the crane but was talking and moving. Phil's colleague gave me the hospital's name and told me to meet him there. An accident, what kind of accident? The crane operator was very upset, and when he called me, he kept repeating that Phil got "jammed up." He was clearly shattered by the incident but tried to explain that Phil got sandwiched between his crane and a cement can.

"Is it serious?"

"He is moving and is talking. I'm so sorry, Julie."

I assumed he had broken some bones; my initial reaction was concern, and it never occurred to me that this was a life-or-death situation. Serious didn't begin to cover it. Just as I was pulling into the emergency room, another call came in on my mobile phone. The hospital social worker asked if I knew how serious the accident was, and she told me she would meet me in the parking lot. When I got out of my car, the social worker rushed over to me, pulled me by the hand, and ran me through the emergency room and into Phil's room. That's when I was told that Phil was in critical condition and was going in for emergency surgery. Phil bled out in the ambulance. His torso, from the neck down, had shattered in five places. He was dead upon arrival at the hospital. I was raced into the emergency room to say goodbye to him. That's how bad it was. A nurse sat me down at the nurse's station as I almost fainted and told me to call my children in.

The first surgery went well and lasted two hours. The next one lasted six hours, and when we gathered as a family in the waiting room, the surgeon came in at 7:00 p.m. and said, "Is the whole family here?"

That's not what you want to hear. I dropped down into the chair and was certain I was going to be told that Phil didn't make it through surgery. I can still hear his voice and see the look on this face when he asked, "Is the family here?"

Phil was alive, for now, but was put into a medical coma. The doctor told me that out of the 352 patients in the hospital, Phil was the hospital's most critical patient. I remember thinking. *That is an award that I never want to win.* He was moved to the trauma ICU and put in bed #10, the one reserved for the most critical patient in the unit, the bed closest to the operating room. He had two round-the-clock nurses assigned to him. His nurses also asked me if our children had been called in. The next forty-eight hours were critical ones for his survival, and the outlook was very uncertain.

Our two boys and daughter were in shock but handling it as well as could be expected. Not only was their dad's back broken in multiple places, but his lungs were also crushed in the accident. Fortunately for Phil, the spine surgeon was on call and did an amazing job. He fused Phil's spine from T2 to T12, and fortunately for me, the hospital was a teaching one, so I was allowed to be with Phil's medical team whenever they discussed the injury and course of treatment. It was the following morning when I realized how significant the injuries were, and they were still unsure if he was going to live.

But honestly, most of my good fortune came from my extended family. My sister and brother took over my life outside of the hospital so I could focus on Phil. I didn't have to worry about getting our children fed or to practice; I didn't have to worry about anything but Phil—they took care of the rest.

Thank God for family.

I met with the team of doctors every day and set up camp in the ICU waiting room. There was so much uncertainty about his lungs and cognitive impairment—because he arrived at the hospital dead—and whether he would ever walk again. Phil was intubated for thirteen days, so his hands were restrained. After a week, they decided to bring him out of the coma and assess if there was a cognitive impairment. He was alert but unable to speak because of the tubes and heavy pain medicine. His nurse was trying to secure his tube in his nose, and his brother said, "Phil, try and keep your head still for the nurses."

Phil turned his head to his brother and very clearly mouthed, "Fuck you."

That sounds crass, but if you knew Phil, hearing him utter those two words after coming out of the coma were the best two words I ever heard. It gave me a great sigh of relief and was a sign, to us anyway, that he might make it through this. I then turned to the nurses and said, "There is no cognitive impairment; Phil is swearing."

Although there was no apparent brain damage from the accident, Phil was scared. And angry.

"Am I going to die?" he asked me.

The nurses on his floor told me Phil was a fighter, which was good, because they were more used to seeing their patients die rather than live. But Phil was anything but guaranteed to survive. Each passing day without a setback was a blessing, but because he was in the ICU for a very long time, the staff knew they had to get him out of there soon. They worried he might get ICU syndrome, which is a type of psychological syndrome that causes the patient to be anxious, depressed, or even delirious.

I had to give permission for the doctors to perform a tracheotomy if he couldn't breathe on his own when they attempted to remove the ventilator.

At 4:00 a.m., still with restrained hands, Phil managed to tear the ventilator tube out. Because he could not breathe on his own, they had to do an emergency intubation. They would attempt the removal again later that day, and if he couldn't breathe on his own, then the tracheotomy was going to be done. Luckily for Phil, on the second attempt to remove it, he was able to breathe.

The day they removed Phil's ventilator, I had to leave the hospital for a job interview. It was the last place I wanted to be, and it was hard to keep myself together, but I didn't think I had much choice. If Phil was unable to pull through or was unable to walk, how would I support my family?

The injury took place on April 15. By May 1, they had moved him to a residential rehabilitation facility. His doctor told him he would need to spend six months there, but to the surprise of everyone, he was home two weeks later. The medical team had never seen anything like that.

My family was still very actively supporting me when Phil came home. They had side rails installed on his side of the bed, but Phil preferred sleeping in the living room recliner. Some adjustments were made to the bathroom for his convenience, but he walked into the home without assistance.

The constant pain was awful. While in the hospital, he was on fentanyl, ketamine, and Oxycontin. By July, he was still relying heavily on the pain medicine drugs, and I was concerned. They changed his demeanor, and not in a good way. After we discussed this together, Phil went cold turkey on all his pain medication. He's the toughest man I know.

Phil went to physical therapy three times a week, and we saw the improvements with each passing week. He was still in tremendous pain, had a permanent cough, and walking the stairs was difficult. But his goal was to get back to work within a year of the injury accident, so May 15, 2019. His doctors thought he was nuts, but that was Phil. Before the injury, the man hadn't missed a day of work in thirty years.

I'll admit, almost everything went right for Phil and me after I received the fateful call about his accident. The surgeon on duty happened to be the spine surgeon; my siblings sprang into action and handled everything outside of Phil's medical care; despite the severity of the injury, Phil recovered faster than anybody imagined; and that job I interviewed for back in May? I got it.

Maybe it was divine intervention? It was more than a year after the accident that Phil finally told me he saw the light—as in *the light* in heaven. He also told me that he spoke to each one of us while he was up there. I don't know if he's shared this with our kids—that's between them—but all I can say is that I appreciate each and every day we have together, and I take a lot less for granted than I used to.

Nobody expects or plans for disaster, but if God forbid it happens to you, my advice is to always say yes to help, no matter how big or small. Don't try to do this alone. When you're making life-and-death decisions for a loved one, you need to make sure your head is clear—and that means you need to get your rest, too.

Phil went back to work one year to the day after his accident.

And we've never hung up on each other since.

BECAUSE HE GOT SICK

by Mark J. Resnick

At the end of my sophomore year in college, I travelled to Kingston, Jamaica with nine other Fairfield University classmates. This wasn't a vacation; it was a mission volunteer trip. None of us stayed in hotels or even with one another, and even though we had met weekly for eight weeks prior, nothing could have prepared me for those ten days in Jamaica.

My friend Jeff and I were assigned to the Sisters of Charity Home for the Dying. Third world country. Downtown Kingston. Home for the Dying. Two college kids. *What could go wrong?*

The Sisters didn't mince words or waste time with their new recruits and assigned us to take care of Mr. Davis, a new arrival. The man, plucked from the streets not long before we arrived that morning, said nothing. He was old, frail, and void of expression. I avoided his eyes and instead stared at his gnarled, matted, and battered dreadlocks. There was a brief moment in which I wondered about the stories and memories contained within those dreads, but it was quickly erased by fear. More like abject terror.

By *take care of him*, the Sisters meant cut his dreads, strip him naked, then bathe, shave, dress, and feed him. I couldn't do it. I froze. But then Jeff said something to me that I will never forget: "Mark, what would we do if these were our dads?" That's all I needed to hear, and I'm forever grateful for Jeff's compassion and wisdom. It took hours, but we managed to take care of Mr. Davis.

Throughout my short volunteer experience at the Home for Dying, I was given a variety of jobs by the Sisters, including cleaning the floors. As awful as that job was, swashing my clean bucket of water and soap with inches of mixed urine, dirt, and mysterious other matter, in my sandals, by the way— nothing was harder than those first few hours with Mr. Davis. But I never thought of myself as a caregiver during those ten days or ten years following. I was just a volunteer. At the end of the day, I left and went about my business. I swapped stories with my classmates, most of whom were assigned to various schools in Kingston, and took as much away from the experience as I could. Little did I know it would one day prepare me to be an actual caregiver.

***

There were early signs that something beyond age-appropriate forgetfulness was at play with my dad. But we missed them all and he was diagnosed with Alzheimer's in 2014. Had he told us about his memory issues sooner, could I have been more helpful to him? Could we have slowed the disease's trajectory with an experimental drug or trial? Would I have learned his story sooner?

To the best of my knowledge, Alzheimer's or dementia were not present within either side of our families, which only made the uncertainty of the diagnosis more stressful. There was no way to understand how agonizing, gut wrenching, unsettling, and at times, frustrating it would be for all of us. We knew the outcome, of course, as the average life expectancy from initial diagnosis is seven years. We just didn't know what to expect along the way or when the end would come. No matter how much you research or learn about the disease, it can't possibly prepare you for the emotional, mental, and physical pain that comes along with it.

To be brutally honest, I used to pray that God would take him peacefully in his sleep. Often, in fact, as in multiple times a day. That is, until he died— then I prayed to God to hug him one more time.

As the months wore on, and I spent more and more time with my dad, I began to look at his Alzheimer's and our relationship differently. I realized how blessed I was to have had him as my dad. And as strange as it may sound, I was getting to know him better than at any point in my life.

Despite the pain and exhaustion that came along with visiting him daily, I also found myself smiling and laughing with him. A lot. I discovered much more than his humor—I witnessed his kindness, curiosity, and compassion toward the assisted living staff and fellow residents. He inspired me every day. His strength, bravery, and resilience were unmatched. What he endured those last few years was remarkable. I never once heard him whine or complain about his situation. There was never a point where he talked about quitting or giving up.

Observing him up close during his battle with Alzheimer's provided an immeasurable perspective on the type of man he was—and as a result—*who I was.*

My dad spent eleven months in assisted living and eighteen more in a nursing home, and no matter how much work I had on my plate or what was happening in my personal life, visiting my dad always came first. I spent the first hour and a half of my day with him, and even then, I could not wait to see him later that night or the next morning. And even though the joy of seeing him inevitably turned to sadness, and I regularly cried in my car after visits, I knew it was the right thing to do—for both of us. He needed to see me to get through his day, and strangely enough, I needed to see him to get through mine as well.

What I can say for certain, then and now, is that I was supposed to be there for my dad during his greatest need. It was not a choice or consideration that required any thinking on my behalf. I visited him every day because I knew being there was hard for him and because I knew our time together had an expiration—and I was adamant that I would not have any regrets about spending as much time as possible with him before he lost his memory for good.

He did lose his memory, and there were no regrets.

Although I lived under his roof for twenty-two years, played under him as my coach in hockey for many years, and worked directly with him in business for thirteen years, I didn't really know who my dad was. Until he got sick, and I became his caregiver.

Alzheimer's was the impetus for an unrivaled kinship but was not the only blessing. His Alzheimer's inspired me to tell his story and share with my children the life-lessons learned from my dad over the past forty-eight years. Lessons that were right in front of me this entire time but had been forgotten, ignored, or outright dismissed.

I can't say for sure that taking care of Mr. Davis in Jamaica in 1992 was *meant to be* or *happened for a reason*. He'll always be part of my story—you never forget those experiences. You never forget hearing the words, "Mark, what if this was our dad who needed to be taken care of?" And you never forget the feeling of giving freely of your time, energy, and love.

When Dad died in August 2021, seven years after his Alzheimer's diagnosis, I experienced a range of conflicting emotions. My role as a caregiver ended, but so did his suffering. I said my final goodbyes to him in the nursing home but had been saying goodbye to him for years. I grieved the loss of my father and best friend but celebrated his life simultaneously through his obituary and the publishing of *Ten Days With Dad*, and his legacy will exist as long as books are part of this world.

It was my dad's Alzheimer's diagnosis that prompted significant changes to my mindset, priorities, focus, and expectations. It was his Alzheimer's that led me to find my purpose and passion in life and come to peace with my past. And it was his Alzheimer's that allowed me to experience the greatest burden and greatest blessing of my life.

Because he got sick—and I was his caregiver.

Mark J. Resnick is an author, speaker, and entrepreneur. He published his debut book, *Ten Days With Dad*, in March 2022. He currently lives in Walpole, MA with his wife Coleen and three children: Campbell, Erin, and Sean.

THE LAST RIDE

by Debbie Johnson

with Mark J. Resnick

April 2010 was a terrible month. My mom was dying. Mainly from old age, but she also had Leukemia and suffered from the killer of all killers for seniors: loneliness. The week of her passing, my husband Henry was on his way to a doctor's appointment. I shouted after him, "And find out why your hands are shaking!"

Before the week ended, my mom died, and Henry received what essentially was a death sentence—he had Parkinson's. The shaking I hardly noticed was Parkinson's, a disease I had no prior knowledge or familiarity. Either way, it was the beginning of the end, a ten-year battle with a terminal disease.

I had to look it up online. The Mayo Clinic defined it as "a progressive disorder that affects the nervous system and parts of the body controlled by nerves." I skimmed the rest. Neither Henry nor I were too keen on knowing every detail about Parkinson's. We knew there was no cure, but early on, we both decided we were going to carry on with our lives for as long as we could.

And that's just what we did—lived our lives. I had opened a restaurant in 2007 and continued to work seven days a week. Henry continued working the night shift at his sheet metal shop and rode his motorcycle. We went about our business, until we no longer could.

About four years after his diagnosis, Henry had to stop working. The shaking was getting worse, and nobody wants a welder with shaky hands near equipment. He was always so good with his hands, whether at work, around the house, or working on his bike. It was the first major setback for him.

By 2016, six years into his battle with Parkinson's, it was time for him to stop driving. I was the bad guy, the person who had to take away his keys.

Henry was also having trouble using the phone, both with dialing and picking it up. His hands betrayed him yet again.

Partly because his former routine involved working late into the night and partly because of Parkinson's, Henry slept a lot during the day and was awake at night. This would prove to be very difficult for me, as I was on the opposite schedule, running a restaurant during the day and sleeping at night. It got to the point where I had to move upstairs to a separate bedroom so that I could get enough sleep to be productive during the day. I didn't realize that the exhaustion I was feeling was only just beginning.

I sold the restaurant in 2017 to take care of Henry full-time. I gave him the option: I could take care of him, or we could hire someone from the outside. He chose me, and I didn't hesitate. I was used to working long hours, seven days a week, but caring for Henry was by far the hardest job I ever had.

In many ways, Henry was reverting to a child. I had to get him dressed each morning; otherwise, it might take him two hours, and both legs would be in the same pant leg. Henry let me dress him without complaint, but there were many activities in which he fought me tooth and nail.

Putting food into his mouth was a chore, but he didn't want my help. Brushing his teeth agitated him even more than feeding him. Not only did I have to bath him, feed him, and lay out his pills, but I also had to stand there and make sure he took them. Like I said, I was often the "bad guy."

I understood his feelings—or tried to as best as one could without experiencing this disease. Becoming dependent on another person to live is hard to accept. Sometimes, I had to let him do his own thing because he wanted to do it—but also because it was too upsetting to watch him struggle. And sometimes I just wasn't in the mood to fight with him, because the more I tried to do for him, the more upset he got. It would only get harder as time went on. What was even more difficult for me was having nobody to talk to about it. My daughter tried to get me to go to a Parkinson's support group, but I said, "Yeah, I'm not one of those people to sit there and spill my guts."

I did find some relief, however, in a very unexpected way. I read an article in the paper about a place called 110 Fitness, which would become, with its new location in Rockland, MA, "the largest wellness center for people afflicted with Parkinson's and other physical disabilities." I mentioned it to Henry, but he had no interest. I went ahead and made an appointment to visit 110 anyway and dragged him along. He had been spending most of his time at home, and I thought this might be good for him. What did we have to lose?

It was the biggest blessing of this entire journey. 110 Fitness and its owner, Brett Miller, changed our lives. At first, I watched Henry work out from a distance with some of the other caregivers. It was good to hear things like, "I'm glad it's not just me dealing with . . . " but before long, I got tired of it. I didn't want to listen to the depressing stories—the very same ones I was experiencing. That's when I volunteered to "corner" for Brett.

Same as a cornerman for a boxer, my job was to help the gym members— most had Parkinson's or something similar like Alzheimer's—get around the ring. Meaning, get from exercise to exercise, provide motivation, and all-around support in getting a safe workout. Helping them stretch or box with the punching bag—it was wonderful. Sometimes, my partner would say, "I just can't do it," to which I would reply, "Sure you can; just give it a try." Before you know it, he was doing it.

I wasn't Henry's corner, mind you. He was happy to have someone else corner for him. They would banter back and forth, and it was a good change of pace for him. I'll say this: 110 Fitness was a game-changer for us both. It got Henry out of the house and to a place where he could be himself with other people suffering from Parkinson's. As for me, I felt like a million bucks. Helping my "patient" feel better made me feel better too. I knew what he was going through, but I got a different response than the one I got from Henry at home.

Henry looked forward to his gym time at 110. I wish we had found it sooner, but it is what it is. After a member's six-month anniversary at the gym, Brett gives them a certificate. When we got home, Henry started to cry as he thanked me for bringing him there. He never wanted to go, but I pushed him, and I tell you again, it was the best thing for us both.

We went to 110 Fitness until COVID-19 struck. When the gym closed, we never made it back.

By this point in Henry's Parkinson's battle, his hallucinations were getting stronger. Not every Parkinson's victim hallucinates, but Henry most certainly did, especially at night or early in the morning. At first, I put a baby monitor in the bedroom so I could hear him get up. Then I installed a camera, which was synched with my phone. I never told Henry about the camera, but I needed one so I could track his movements at night. It was common to hear the water running late at night, and it was Henry on his hands and knees outside the shower stall, trying to wash himself. Sometimes, he let me coax him back to bed; other times, I was giving him a shower at 3:00 a.m.

It was part of the progression. Unfortunately, Henry was losing his sense of self and surroundings, and I was losing every ounce of energy caring for him. He was also falling more often. He would stand and fall, and then I would pick him up. He had a wheelchair but didn't like using it. The falls continued until one night he got out of bed, and I couldn't get him up. The ambulance took him to the hospital. There were no major injuries, and Henry was alert and speaking to me. He was actually feeling pretty good, considering the late stage of his disease.

That final night in the hospital was our last conversation. I never got anything out of him after he left and moved into a nursing home for three days. When a bed opened up in a nursing home in Rockland, we moved him there, only I had trouble seeing him, as this was during the COVID-19 shutdowns. He was there a week and a half before I saw him.

The disease was taking over, and I agreed to sign papers for hospice to care for him. Before leaving for the night, I kissed him goodbye and said, "See you in the morning." Even though hospice was now on sight, I didn't feel like it was the end. He could no longer speak to me, but his eyes were open. Nobody gave me a timeline or warning that this might be the end. There was no "he only has a few days left" announcement from anybody.

Henry died the following morning.

It still eats at me because had I known it was the end, I would have stayed with him that night. It only reinforced my nagging thoughts of how I "failed" Henry. I know this isn't true or fair of me to judge myself so harshly, but I did, at least for a while.

In March, I went back to 110 Fitness. Henry was no longer with me, but I longed for community—the 110 Community. It was a positive place. A home. I had retired early to care for Henry, but I'm only sixty-four years old. I need something to do and have always been a worker. I'm comfortable there and know I am helping others face this cruel disease. I know what they're going through.

In order to return to 110, I had to take a job at night, which I gladly did. This allows me to work four days a week, either at the gym or pool. Parkinson's is awful, but if I can help put a smile on someone's face, even for just a few hours a week, I feel like I am doing something good.

I miss Henry every day. I don't miss the day-to-day caregiving part because it was the hardest thing I've ever had to do in my life. But it also made me a better wife—a better person. I became a little more patient. I tried my best to make him happy and to make his life easier.

In 2019, when he wanted to see his friends and family one last time, I took him on a 4,000-mile trip to four states. Parts of the trip were hell. I drove from MA to North Carolina to see our daughter—sixteen hours straight. Then to Florida to see Smitty, his lifelong buddy. Henry knew it was the last time they would see each other, and although he didn't talk much—because he couldn't communicate what he wanted to say—he enjoyed himself. I could feel that he was happy.

From Florida, I drove to Tennessee, then back to North Carolina, then back home. Always driving straight through. We couldn't stay at a hotel because of how he behaved—I didn't want people to think I was abusing him. It was an eighteen-day marathon down, up, and over the East Coast. It wasn't easy, but we managed, and I was happy that Henry got to say goodbye to the people he loved.

I did the best I could. I took the brunt of his frustration. I was the bad guy who took his car and motorcycle away from him. I had to say "no" more often than I cared to. I had to help him eat and brush his teeth, and so much more. I cleaned up more messes in a day before most people had their morning coffee.

People asked me all the time how Henry was doing. They never asked how the caregiver was doing. It was upsetting at times. I couldn't tell people what it was like—what I was going through. I sat down and recorded my thoughts in a journal each day, just to have someone or something to talk to. It was a way to release my anger without unloading on someone. I recommend trying this to any caregiver that will listen to me.

There's no room for regrets or second-guessing myself.

I must be doing some good for the 110 Community, as Brett honored me at his recent fundraising Gala as Volunteer of the Year. I despise attention and didn't want the recognition, but in a way, I needed it. It validated what I was doing with my time and focus, helping families and patients live with Parkinson's.

As Henry rides his bike on the roads of Heaven, hands no longer shaking, I know he's smiling. I know he's proud of me for staying in the fight on behalf of others, whether as a corner woman, Parkinson's advocate, or friendly face to someone in need.

Debbie Johnson is a retired restaurant owner. She has called Weymouth home since the late 70's when she and her husband, Henry, settled after marrying. She found 110 to be the community she and Henry needed when they took on the challenges Parkinson's threw their way. Even after losing Henry, she finds strength in the community and continues the work at 110 by volunteering as a corner person. The work is rewarding and gives her as much strength as she hopes to share with others.

THERE'S NO CURE FOR PTSD

by Susan Tallman

with Mark J. Resnick

I've been a pharmacy technician for twenty-five years, and most of the time, I love my job. Living in a medium-sized city, I get to know people on a personal level. I see the "regulars" who have chronic illnesses, allergies, or conditions, but there's a fair amount of people who come into the pharmacy for the first time—at least for the first time with a serious need for medication. I never thought my interactions with customers, both old and new, would help me become a better caregiver for my husband, Ron, but it has.

I don't know what the definition of a caregiver is; I never thought much about it until I was asked to share my caregiving story for this book. Ron doesn't have any physical injuries and hasn't been diagnosed with a disease that might kill him. He had colon cancer and still has a pacemaker, which was installed in 2021, but there are no obvious signs that he needs any care whatsoever.

Ron's wounds aren't physical—they're mental. His wounds run deeper than any I've ever seen or heard about.

Ron and I met in Chester, OH, at a Civil War enactment. Ron was a participant, and I was a volunteer (actually, my brother "volunteered" me to help at the event, and I'm glad he did)! Later that evening, I met Ron at the bar, and we connected right away. After the weekend, we kept in touch by phone and visited one another a few times. We married in 2007.

I knew Ron was a Vietnam veteran. He signed up for the army at age nineteen and was deployed to Vietnam shortly after. During his second year of duty, he suffered a physical injury and was sent home. The injury was physical, and he healed, but he's been emotionally wounded since the day he came home, like thousands of others who fought in the war.

Ron's proud of his service on behalf of his country, and he remains a big part of celebrating veterans to this day. He and others from the VFW, American Legion, and Elks organize Memorial Day parades and guest speakers. But Ron also carries with him enormous guilt, anger, and trauma. He's not proud of what happened in Vietnam—of what he and so many other young kids were asked to do. It haunts me just listening to him speak about it.

My father was a World War II veteran, and I know he and Ron spoke often about their respective services. Unlike my dad, Ron was a disaster when he returned home from combat. It took years for him to function like a "normal" young man—to be able to wake up with purpose, find a job, and work toward a future.

For twenty-five years, Ron managed stores for Aubuchon Hardware. His battle with colon cancer forced him to retire, but by the time we met, he was already in remission. He calls himself retired, but he's active with his carpentry and volunteering. Sitting still has never been easy for him, and part of me wonders if that has anything to do with his PTSD. I know I wouldn't want too much alone time had I even a fraction of the thoughts that consume his mind.

Veterans with PTSD are not always in rough shape. Ron goes for extended periods of time without needing to see a VA counselor or open up to me. The difficult aspect of the condition is that you never know when it will strike. It could be a scene from a movie, fireworks, or the time of year. For example, March is Vietnam Veterans Month, so that's a tough time for him. PTSD never goes away.

The VA network has been good for Ron. There are times when he'll say, "Maybe I should make an appointment to talk to someone." And I'll say, "Yes, I think you should." Listening to Ron is my biggest strength and duty as his caregiver, but he needs somebody else to talk to besides me.

When I listen to Ron, I become sad and teary-eyed. It's difficult to listen to what he tells me, to comprehend why they were asked to do certain tasks.

"I don't understand why I'm still here," he would say.

The survivor's guilt is enormous. I sit, listen, console, and listen some more. I don't have to answer him or ask questions or suggest anything. I listen and show him compassion. I hate to see him during these rough patches. It was like this recently. After work one night, I questioned whether or not I should call in sick and stay with him the next day, but he wanted me to go to work. This happens at least four times a year.

It just makes me very sad, hearing things that happened over there, what he had to take part in. It does affect me, but I need to be the strong one and listen to what he has to say. That's where the pharmacy experience has helped. It's my job to listen and be compassionate. To help them through whatever it is that they are dealing with, at least with the complicated insurance coverage innuendos.

In addition to the VA, the VFW has been a safe place for Ron all these years. I never knew how powerful and supportive the VFW was across the country. I knew nothing about the programming they do locally and nationally. When a veteran struggles to pay a bill, they jump in. It's so much more than a social spot for them to connect and support one another.

Getting him through his depression periods is the hardest part for me. Like I said, I never know when they are coming. He talks more now than he ever did, which is really good. Usually late night. But whether it takes an hour or all night long, I sit and listen.

There are some things about his past in Vietnam that he won't discuss. And when he's sleeping, you don't want to wake him up or touch him because he might wake up and be ready to fight. This is a frequent occurrence and something that upsets me, too.

I know for Ron, helping other veterans has been so helpful for his own healing. He has spoken to soldiers returning from Iraq and Afghanistan. He got one young man into the VA for help, and he often reaches out to Ron to thank him for doing that.

If you're in this situation, whether someone's trauma is combat-related or not, my advice is to take your time. Don't rush the person who needs your help. Meet them where they are. Encourage them to get help and get them to the right places, but it takes time and patience. Believe me, they don't want to have this problem.

PTSD never goes away, but we can try to ease the pain by listening and getting our loved ones the help and support they need.

DANCING WITH MOM

by Lynda Starr-Zimmerman
with Mark J. Resnick

My mom, Ruth Starr, was diagnosed with dementia at eighty-four, though she likely suffered from the disease well before the formal diagnosis. Our first big clue that she might have dementia was after a birthday dinner for my son Cameron.

Despite her age, Mom was still driving, and after sharing "goodbyes" and "I love yous" with each other, she got in her car and prepared to drive herself home. My husband Joe, daughter Mandy, and I did the same. It was past 8:00 p.m., and traffic was light, but instead of turning onto her lane heading north toward home, she crossed over the divider and drove on the wrong side of the road, directly at incoming traffic. It was scary, but we somehow followed her and turned her around, and she got home safely.

My mom was the baby in her family. Her older sister had dementia, and we sometimes worried mom might be heading there as well. It became extremely worrisome when she almost got herself killed driving that night. Mom was living by herself at the time. Before the diagnosis, I remember going to her apartment and seeing that her refrigerator was scarce yet full of outdated foods. She wore the same clothes almost every time we saw her and struggled to take her medications consistently. Shortly after, a doctor confirmed her dementia diagnosis. It was time for her to give up her apartment and come to live with us. My brother, sister, and I agreed to share responsibility and alternate caring for our mom.

The plan was to have Mom live with my brother Mitch in Boston during the week, then alternate weekends living with my sister and me. The arrangement seemed fine at first, until it wasn't. None of us could take her in full-time because of existing family circumstances. It became clear over time that the disruption of her routine was too much for her, causing confusion and stress. Knowing what I now know about the disease, I realize her condition was probably exasperated by the constant moving from home to home, as people with dementia crave familiarity and routine.

There were many challenges caring for my mom during the four years she lived with us. We never felt like we could give her the proper care she needed and deserved. My mom became very agitated if we didn't give her 100% of our attention, making it difficult to cook, clean, or do simple tasks like sorting the mail and paying bills. Then there were the outbursts, which got out of control at times, leaving us feeling worried and unsure of what to do. Her dementia was a very trying time for all of us, and I wish there was more guidance and support for family members to learn how to best care for their loved ones in these situations.

I enjoyed having Mom with me those weekends, but in addition to my full-time job, I also had a part-time job as a bartender. There were some Sundays I had to work, so Joe would take my mom to visit me at the restaurant for a few hours to break up the day and be around other people. One time, she said to Joe, "That's really nice that you still wear your wedding ring, even though your wife is dead." My husband said to me, "Bad news, Lynda. Ruthie killed you off." My mom thought she was on a date with my handsome husband. Mom was a feisty one. In fact, her high school yearbook quote was "Gigantic Sauciness." And saucy she was.

One morning, Joe and I were lying in bed, getting ready to start the day. My mom knocked on our bedroom door and peaked her adorable, 4'10" little self in and said, "Is the lady going to make breakfast?" Ruth thought she was in a hotel—and to this day, Joe still thinks it's hilarious to refer to me as the breakfast or lunch lady. He often says, "Has anybody seen the lunch lady? She is late?"

Joe has a vivid memory of my mom's realization of how old she was. Joe was driving her home from an event, when they began a discussion of how old her children were. She guessed that I was twenty-five (I was actually fifty-five; thanks, Mom). She looked in the mirror with hands pressed up against

162

her face and said in disbelief, "If she's fifty-five, how the heck old am I?" She was mortified to see her image in the mirror.

Around the time when my mom was turning ninety, my brother had to have emergency eye surgery. My sister-in-law was able to get my mom into a room at the Marion Manor Nursing Home in South Boston. It was a temporary visit due to Mitch's surgery, but shortly after, a room opened up full-time at the Sherrill House in Boston, which was both a nursing home and rehab center. It became her permanent home until she died at the age of ninety-eight.

The nursing home was such a blessing. It was clean, and the care in the dementia unit was good. She was safe, and you could tell she felt that way too. Mom's memory was pretty much gone when she lived with us, and the disease progressed in the nursing home. She would get worse sometimes when dealing with an illness or adjustment to her medications. Her last glimmers of recognition of me—of any of her family—were about a year into her stay at Sherill House. Unfortunately, for most of the time in the nursing home, she didn't really know who we were. On occasion, she would refer to me as her baby, and it made me so happy.

But in reality, it was a very long, slow goodbye to my mom.

Mom lost her memory, but she maintained her joyful personality throughout most of her stay in the nursing home. She was known for always singing and dancing at every opportunity. Even toward the end of her life, she still hummed songs.

We knew my mom struggled to remember much, and COVID-19 did even more damage to her short-term memory. She got COVID-19 twice and survived despite her heart disease. Recreation time was eliminated, which meant her singing and dancing were too. She was confined to her room, and without regular visits from family and social interactions with other residents, her dementia worsened at warp speed. We tried to speak to her through Zoom calls, but she struggled to focus, and the calls didn't last long. Often, we would just sing together. The calls become more depressing than uplifting—the joy had disappeared—for everyone.

By the time we could visit her again, her disease had progressed immensely. Her communication was nearly nonexistent; she was confined to a wheelchair, and she spent most of her time in bed. She could still hum, and I knew it brought her joy right until the very end of her life.

As people get dementia, they are often forgotten—who they were, what they did, and what their passions were. We must not forget. My mom was once so full of life. She was very involved in her synagogue and served as its president, where she gave many thoughtful and inspiring speeches. She was also involved in her community and in our family. She was a singer, dancer, and portrait artist. My mom was glamorous, lively, and confident. For many years, she volunteered to be a crossing guide, only she insisted she was a "police lady." She was so proud of her responsibility. We found it cute and amusing that she referred to herself as the police lady.

We held a very small funeral for my mom. At the age of ninety-eight, she had outlived her friends and her five siblings. Just immediate family were in attendance. It was perfect.

We played a couple of her favorite songs at the funeral, songs that would help move her soul—to dance her way into the heavens. Frank Sinatra was one of her favorites, so we played *Gimme Me A Little Kiss* and *A Your Adorable* before the ceremony started. I held up my iPhone and played it softly but loudly enough for all to hear and sing along.

That's when I felt it. All of a sudden, I got the urge to dance. You have to understand—I am not a dancer. I don't dance, and I don't like to be the center of attention. But something came over me. I grabbed Mitch and Harlene, my siblings, and we danced. I went through the small gathering of family and danced with them all—some reluctantly, but doing it to honor my mom—as they smiled with confusion. I felt like my mom had taken over my body. It was an odd yet joyful sensation to dance with my mom at her funeral.

When the singing and dancing ended, the Rabbi said, "I have officiated thousands of funerals in my life, and this was definitely a first! That was so beautiful. What a way to honor your mom."

"It wasn't me," I replied. "That was my mom!"

Hope you are dancing in heaven with one of your two husbands or maybe your longtime boyfriend.

Dance in peace, Mom.

FINDING PURPOSE AS A CAREGIVER

by *Vicki Langevin*

Care·giv·er /ˈkerˌɡivər/*noun*

- a family member or paid helper who regularly looks after a child, sick, elderly, or disabled person.

When I read this vague definition of "caregiver," I never imagined that one day I could give it a thousand more detailed, raw, precious, and heart-wrenching meanings. I never signed up to be a caregiver. I would have laughed if you had told me that someday I would take on this role, and yet, I was my father's caregiver for the last five years of his life.

My father and I had our ups and downs while I was growing up. I wasn't the most well-behaved teenager in the world, and with five other siblings to contend with for attention, Dad had his hands full. If one of us were disobedient, all Mom had to say was, "You wait until your father gets home!" With that one statement, I did my best to behave; I just wasn't always successful. But as life went on, we grew up and eventually put it all behind us.

My parents divorced as I neared adulthood. Afterward, Dad lived alone. He maintained his small house, did his own chores, worked the local bingo halls, and continued on at the warehouse where he had worked for more than forty years. I checked in on Dad often, either in person, on the phone, or at whichever bingo hall he was working. He was an independent person and often jovial when he was out in public—but privately, he was a loner. It was this side of my dad that made it hard to get to know him growing up.

Nur·ture /ˈnərCHər/*noun*
- the process of caring for and encouraging the growth or development of someone or something.

As my father and I began to foster our adult child/parent relationship, I began to notice some changes in his behavior. He had trouble with some of the little things, like not remembering how to use the TV remote or misplacing his house or car keys. During my check-ins, he would be sitting in his rocking chair, doing a word search with a little handheld radio playing beside him. He'd explain the problem, and I would fix it or try to accommodate his requests. I always reminded him to call me right away if he needed help. For the lost keys, we decided to always place them in a glass candy dish on the bare kitchen table.

"I'm fine, I promise," he would say before I left the house.

This was the beginning of me jumping into my caregiver role headfirst, uneducated, helpless, and unprepared for what was to come. As things continued to unravel, I began accompanying Dad to his doctor appointments. I was with him when he received the diagnosis: Alzheimer's disease. A progressive monster that destroys memory and other mental functions, slowly or quickly, over time. Nothing could have prepared my father, a hard-working and independent man, for all he was about to lose—or me, as his sole provider.

Life was a constant ebb and flow, going from calm to crazy in a moment. I had to re-adapt Dad to his surroundings on a daily basis, which required a level of creativity on my part to make his life livable and independent. This may seem simple, but it is heartbreaking to witness and be part of. I had to take over every aspect of my father's life—caring for him, managing his schedule, keeping him safe, feeding, clothing, and medicating him safely. His entire existence was now my responsibility. There was never a question that this was to be my role, and there was never any doubt that I could and would wholeheartedly do this for him.

Com·pan·ion /kəmˈpanyən/*noun*

- a person or animal with whom one spends a lot of time or with whom one travels.

Dad was stubborn. He made excuses for not being able to do certain tasks by acting like he just didn't have the time. I had to read between the lines and hear what wasn't said in order to manage his symptoms without him feeling humiliated. He tried hard to hide his decline from me, and I tried hard, in turn, to pretend I didn't see his struggle.

The single most defining moment in this new father-daughter relationship was when I realized that he didn't recognize me anymore. He would ask me if he was my first patient or my last for the day. He wanted to know if I had kids, if I was married, and if I grew up around Barre. A few times, he asked who my parents were—maybe he knew them.

I was always honest with him that he was my father, and my mother was Barb, but he never believed it.

Dad still lit up and smiled when I arrived with his morning coffee and burritos from McDonald's, probably because I had food. He listened as I told him the weather prediction, what to expect for the coming days, when I would be back to check on him, and what was for lunch. I scheduled Meals on Wheels deliveries as an extra eye and a friendly face. I would leave childproof scissors so he could open his own snack packages and prepare his drinks for him to grab in the fridge. I made it easy for him to get about his home during the day.

Even though he had no recollection of our former relationship as father and daughter, he recognized me as a person who cared for him, loved him, watched over him, and would be there for him whenever he needed something. He could count on me. It hurt for a while, but eventually, I was okay with this. "Daughter" was my old title. It brought me peace that he felt safe and confident in knowing me as his "friend."

I never imagined how many times I would have to lie to my father just so he wouldn't get hurt or upset. One of the lies I told the most concerned his own parents. He thought they were still alive. He would ask me if I had seen them that day.

"Yes, Dad, I stopped and saw them on my way here. They weren't feeling well today, but your mom said she would try to come by tomorrow."

In hindsight, I feel I did the right thing, protecting him and keeping him from pain. I also used to have to tell him I would give him a ride home when I was done working on days when he didn't think he was in his own home and wanted to go "home." Those days were hard, just knowing he was excited to finally go back home. Some days, he would have forgotten by the time I got there after work. Other days, he would be packed, ready, and waiting for me. On those days, I didn't know if it would take one hour or four to talk him down, get him supper, and get him settled for the night. Each day was different and unique.

Fa·ther / ˈfäTHər/*noun*
- a man in relation to his child or children.

In the fall of 2020, in the thick of the pandemic, Dad had to go to the hospital for a week and then into "rehab" at a local nursing home. At that time, visitors were not allowed into the facility. It was a hard time for me. I worried so much about him being away from me, with no real one-on-one care like he was accustomed to. I had been at the helm of his daily life, keeping him safe and grounded for years, and now I couldn't even see him.

To cope, I focused on making his home safer and more feasible for him to remain independent. My family painted, moved furniture, secured the TV to a stand on the wall, bought a new recliner, organized his clothing, moved his bed out to the living room, installed cameras (watching his every move from an iPad set up at my home childcare business), and built a big gated and covered deck—the list goes on and on.

Once Dad's legs healed, he was released back to my care safely. The day I got him out of the facility and brought him home was a wonderful one until later that night, he started to cry and told me he wanted me to bring him home. It was a punch in the gut after all I had done, but more so because he really didn't recognize his own home where he had lived for more than twenty years.

I managed as best I could to stay one step ahead of my dad's decline by putting a gate on the deck so he wouldn't fall down the stairs, buying him pants with an elastic waistband, packing away his button-down shirts because he couldn't button, zip, or do his belt buckle anymore; and getting his night-time ice cream bowl ready ahead of time in the freezer with a spoon because he no longer could. I made life as easy as I could for him to navigate. These simple changes also made my job easier for me in the long run. Just like he had in the beginning of all this, he would avoid doing things that he wasn't sure how to do, like opening containers, making phone calls, or changing the channel. The list got longer as time marched on.

Love /ləv/*verb*
* feel deep affection for (someone).

Caring for him was a task that changed daily. I had to devise new ways to do just about everything. His pill administration went from him taking care of it himself to me taping a large calendar to the kitchen counter to remind him when to take them to me keeping his pills in pill cases that I administered (he would check the days off for me), to me bringing him all his pills in daily. Sometimes, he would obsess over his pills, so I would leave empty bottles in the cupboard. That seemed to leave him reassured that he still had some control over his own life. Having done this for himself all his life, he must have struggled to hand it over to someone else.

When I first committed to caring for my father, I knew that I wouldn't have the support of my siblings and accepted it. I was glad to not consult with anyone regarding his care; there were no schedules to update for his care, and no arguing about it either. My partner, Scott, would go to my dad's at a moment's notice to help him with anything. My mother would also wash, dry, and fold Dad's laundry every week at her house. And I had a tribe of children who would stop in and check on Dad as needed. I am very grateful for these people who supported me and my dad as best they could.

Daugh·ter /ˈdôdər/*noun*
• a girl or woman in relation to either or both of her parents.

At the beginning of my caregiving journey, I had a list of a few things that I swore I would never do for my father. I said I would never help my dad shower. Nope, I did not want to see my father naked. But he needed me, and I was there for him, no matter what. Those moments were very humbling. In times when Dad's mind was sharp, he would cry, saying that these were not things that a daughter should have to do for her father. I made it clear to him that I didn't mind helping him and that I loved him very, very much. I loved when he was all freshly showered and feeling good about himself.

There were also times when his disease took over, and he would say things that no daughter should ever have to hear—times that were hard to swallow and left me unsettled for days. I told myself if he ever had an "accident," I would not be the one to clean it up. But those times were when he needed me the most. He needed me, and I needed to be the one to help him. Did I do these things for him? Absolutely. Every time.

Heart /härt/*noun*
• the central or innermost part of something.

I am glad that he trusted me enough to hand it all over to me, or maybe I just took it over because it was the right thing to do at the moment. I loved my father so much; I can't imagine turning my back the other way when he needed me the most. I would never have had any of these clarifying moments had I not stepped in and taken over the small details he was missing in the beginning of his Alzheimer's battle.

Caring for my father cost me time with my own six children and my four grandchildren. I was so invested in my father's care and well-being that I had no time for anything else, and I had no backup to fill my shoes if I needed or wanted a break. I lost minutes, hours, days, and months with them that I can't get back. This was the ultimate price to pay for what I did for my father. My one hope is that I have set an example for my children through the sacrifices I made in caring for my father the way I did.

In being the eyes, ears, and voice for my dad, I had to make many decisions on his behalf. In a sense, I almost had to be him and imagine what he would do or want done. I hope each decision I made was the right one, and I hope I made him proud of me. At first, I had a hard time making choices for him, small and large—being "the boss," as we used to joke. Once it was very clear he was incapable of this task, I became a fierce advocate for him. I cannot imagine what would have happened to my father if he hadn't had someone on his side, in his corner, looking out for him with love and care.

Unfortunately, in the last year of his life, my father got violent with me. It started when he had a strange week filled with very odd behaviors, and it ended with him hitting, slapping, pushing, and biting me. He had no idea if I was his daughter, friend, caretaker, or stranger. There's a part of me that wonders what he saw that night—but I can't let it consume me because we will never know. I had been in contact with his doctor during that week and had asked what I should do if his behavior progressed. I was told to bring him to the Emergency Department for admission and get him on some psych meds for his behavior. I didn't like the advice, but I kept it in mind.

The day after he attacked me, I admitted him to the hospital where he stayed from May through September. I was there every night to help him eat dinner, change his clothes, and get him settled for the night. The hospital tested him and tried med changes to get him to a point where he could function without aggression. The hospital ended up placing my father in a nursing facility three and a half hours away from me. I never felt more helpless and scared. Helpless because it was me against the hospital and insurance company and scared because he was so very far away from me, and I couldn't be there for or with him.

While he was there, I was able to visit a few times, and we did video calls where I could see and talk to him. But I was also fighting hard to get him back home and advocating for him every minute that he was away from me. After a month, I got him into a private home in Williamstown through the Choice Program, where he was the only other resident and would basically have one-on-one care—and I could see him anytime I wanted.

I joyfully got him all set up at his new place on October 11, 2021. I was able to get him his McDonald's favorites and his peanut butter and jelly sandwiches. I brought his favorite things from his own home, including his robotic cat, family photos, his blankets, pillows, and clothing.

He was close enough that I was able to see him every night after I got done working. I was able to meet with Home Health and his therapy nurse team. My father was put on hospice care after he had only been back a few days. Nearing the end of Dad's second week at his new place, before I left for the night, I put his wedding ring back on his left ring finger. Years ago, he had told me that he wanted to be buried with his wedding ring on, despite the fact that my parents had divorced years ago. A promise is a promise, Dad. I got back to my home just in time to answer the ringing phone. Dad had taken a turn and wasn't expected to last through the night. I drove back to him immediately.

I had my precious father back with me for twelve whole days before he went to Heaven on October 23. In a candlelit room, with Ann Murray softly playing next to his ear from my phone, holding his hands, watching his eyebrows rise and fall at the sounds from here and beyond all around him, listening to his uneven, untimely breaths and telling him how much I loved him, he slipped away from me.

The only words to describe that surreal moment in time were "deafening," "awful," and "scary." My father, who I had focused my life on helping to this point, was gone. No one can prepare you for this. Not only had I lost my father, but I had also lost my purpose, my drive, my person. What would I do without him? How would I proceed?

The next minutes, hours, days, and months are now just a blur to me. So many things to do, things to settle, and paperwork to fill out. It was a trying time, for sure. Through it all, one wish prevailed. My wish for my father was that when he reached the heavenly gates, all the memories he had forgotten—big and small, good and bad, happy and sad—would come flooding back to him.

Prior to my father's death, when he was in the nursing facility three hours away, a friend asked me to help provide care for her elderly uncle, who had begun to show signs of dementia and had just lost his wife. "Of course," I said. "Absolutely. When do I start?"

I figured it would help keep my mind busy while my own dad was so far away, and I missed caring for someone and helping them, so why not. I am still caring for this gentleman today, almost a year and a half later, and I am able to fill the hole in my heart left by the loss of my own dad. I cook his dinner and spend a good chunk of time with him five nights a week, helping him navigate, staying one step ahead, and sharing a lot of laughs together along the way.

Though I once scoffed at the thought of caring for anyone—let alone my dad—it is now my purpose and passion. I can't imagine my life without serving as a caregiver.

Vicki Langevin is a mother, grandmother, daughter, sister, aunt, friend and dog mom. She writes for fun and therapy, loves crafts, puzzles, and cooking. A child of the 70's faced with raising her parents, she takes on the role with grace and grit. She lives in Central Vermont with her family and dogs Marcie and Charlie.

MAYBE IT WILL GO AWAY

by Janet Steward

The Devil Dogs were the worst, with their chocolate-colored, sawdust-textured outer layer that sandwiched a white, whipped, sugary middle layer. My nose turned up when one of those plastic-wrapped torpedoes greeted me upon opening my Cinderella lunchbox. Twinkies were not much better. A flat-bottomed golden sponge cake, they were filled with a similar sugary white fluff.

My favorites were the Hostess chocolate cupcakes, which came two to a package. The chocolate frosting, hardened into a flat cap, which could be peeled off while still intact. Bisecting that dark frosting was a firm, squiggly line of white fondant. Just one or two bites into the moist chocolate cake brought crumb-crusted lips to the middle of the cupcake, where the whipped sugary center awaited.

When I was a child and young adolescent, the snack drawer was filled with a Hostess potpourri. We were allowed to choose one dessert to add to our school lunch, carefully arranged within the square tin box and lunchbox-themed thermos.

One day in 1965, the snack drawer was empty. Not one cupcake, Twinkie, or Devil Dog to be found. Not even a Ding Dong. My brother Charlie and I were redirected to the refrigerator to pack our lunch—the crisper drawer now replete with fresh apples, oranges, and pears.

It was a sudden change for sure, but giving up the Twinkie drawer turned out to be not so bad. Instead, the house began filling with the heady and intoxicating aroma of freshly baked bread. Tender sourdough bread, dense molasses and cornmeal-crusted Anadama bread, tangy Swedish rye laced with caraway seeds, and mouthwatering oatmeal and honey whole wheat bread.

This happened right after my mother visited the Goddard College Adult Degree Program in Vermont. Long before becoming popular and trendy, my mother made the conscious decision to consume only organic foods, whole wheat, no sugar, and no red meat. Not only did she decide to *eat* healthy, but she also made a commitment to *be* healthy. Growing up in Alabama, she had learned to swim early and enjoyed it as recreation. At the age of forty, swimming became a passion and daily activity for my mother, receiving her 1000-mile swim badge several times over.

It's hard to argue against the logic of eating healthy, but the visit to Vermont did not change my mother in the manner that mattered most: how she treated me as her daughter. My mother saw a daughter as a threat and competition for my father's affection. She spent my entire life trying to convince my father—and me—that I was worthless, selfish, and greedy. But I was a kid. I did not know there could be anything but the neglect and disdain I endured growing up. In my family, I was taught I was never good enough. And I believed it.

But meeting Bob changed everything. We both had deep emotional scars and hearts that had been badly broken. We fell madly in love and discovered that unconditional love can truly heal broken hearts. Bob and I felt so lucky and blessed to have found each other and looked forward to spending the rest of our lives together. Finally, I was good enough. Everything seemed perfect.

Until 1993.

"Bring me a pair of gloves, will you?" Bob called from the bathroom addition he was building in the spring of 1993. "My hands are kind of sore."

Bringing him a pair of blue-felted "monkey gloves," I examined his hands—hands well-accustomed to physical labor and hard work. They were thickly muscled and calloused from milking cows as a child on his grandparents' farm and cutting timber as a teenager with a crosscut. As an adult, those hands ran skidders and chainsaws, and they planted, hilled, and harvested fields of Green Mountain potatoes. Having taught welding, mechanics, and building trades as the Chair of the Industrial Arts Department, Bob's well-worked hands were now raw, skin peeling off in sheets.

"Must be from handling these hemlock studs," he said as I grimaced, looking at his hands. The golden beams smelled of pitch and softwood glades. "When I finish framing the walls, maybe it will go away."

The completed addition was everything we had hoped for, with walls paneled in smooth knotty pine boards Bob had logged and sawn, a shower and bubbly hot tub installed, and large-paned windows offering an expansive view of fields and mountains. With the new bathroom finished, Bob began removing the tiny original bathroom to enlarge the kitchen, hands still raw and gloved as he tore out dusty bathroom walls and the sage-green sink, toilet, and tub.

Now, under his dark green Dickey's pants, Bob's legs were red, raw, and itchy, shedding skin in concert with his hands.

"Maybe it's the detergent I have been using," I mused, thinking of the perfumed scent. "I'll try a different one—maybe it will go away." Changing laundry detergent had no effect on the spreading, pervasive, and unpleasant symptoms Bob experienced. He consented to see a doctor, hoping for a simple solution to make the symptoms go away. Allergy tests, colloidal oatmeal, cold showers, warm baths, prescription creams, and ointments all had no effect.

Bob was now alternately freezing cold or sweating profusely, as if his internal thermostat had gone haywire.

Turning onto the off-ramp of Exit 20 on I-89S, we parked, and with trepidation, we scuffed along the curved, gray cement pathway through the double doors, wondering what lay ahead. Sitting on the cold, hard metal examining table, clothed in nothing but a thin blue Johnnie, Bob racked with shivers. The room smelled of antiseptic and floor polish. While he was being examined by the head of the dermatology department, a steady stream of interns entered the room.

With smooth rubber-gloved hands and starched white coats that swished as they moved, the interns manipulated every inch of Bob. Their fingers slid quickly, then slowly, then quickly again from the top of Bob's head to the bottoms of his feet. Rubber-encased fingers touched raised red lesions, scaly skin, and peeling patches. With lips pursed and brows furrowed, the interns whispered to each other, their pens rapidly scratching notes on narrow-ruled pads.

Watching, I wanted to scream, "He is a person, not an object to be poked and pried." But I remained silent, hoping that suffering this indignity would bring answers to make the painful and disturbing symptoms go away.

With Bob's flaking and reddened back exposed, the interns crammed closer, craning their necks as the dermatologist's shiny scalpel sliced a slug-shaped and sized sample from a raised scaly patch just below Bob's right shoulder. The bloody blob dropped silently onto a petri dish. The doctor deftly stitched up the incision, alternating between poking the threaded needle and pulling it tight while whispers wafted and pens scratched.

Turning to Bob, the doctor said, "You may get dressed now. We'll be in touch soon."

Exiting the examining room, the doctor was followed by a parade of swishing, white-coated interns who were gesturing and speaking softly among themselves.

Left alone in the examining room, Bob and I glanced at each other, trying to cheer each other up with a hopeful, "Maybe it will go away."

A week later, while teaching first grade, I was summoned to the office for a telephone call. "It's the Dermatology Department at Dartmouth." My breath catching, my feet waged war with themselves, wanting to both run to the phone and not take one step toward what I feared might be unwelcome news.

"Is this Mrs. Steward?" the saccharine voice on the other end inquired. "This is the dermatology department. I believe your husband was in last week for a biopsy."

I squeezed out a barely audible, "Yes."

"We have the results of Mr. Steward's tests. He has cutaneous T-cell lymphoma."

Trying to portray some semblance of calm, I asked, "Can you repeat that?" Then I added, "What does that mean?"

Her words traveled again through the receiver. "Cutaneous T-cell lymphoma. He has cancer. He might live three years; he won't live five."

The office's wooden shelf, laden with frayed telephone books, spiral-bound memo books, crisp white and colored copying paper, and sundry school supplies, held me up as I fell against it, eyes tightly shut to block out what I had just heard.

Cancer. Bob, fifty-four years old, I, forty-two. Although teachers are not supposed to be the ones crying at school, I wailed and sobbed uncontrollably as if my heart was breaking.

It was, and it did.

The man who had saved me from insecurity, loneliness, and so much pain from a life before him—a life without love and affirmation from my mother—was dying. And so was I. A piece of me died with Bob, who made it three—but not five years.

Maybe the heartache will go away, I thought. It did not. Although over time, I have learned to survive and even live without Bob in my life, the intensity of those tears and pain echoed the love we shared. I don't ever want that to go away.

Ten years after Bob's passing, I was called upon to be a caregiver again—this time, for someone who had never given me the love I had been blessed to receive from Bob. It was not until after Bob died that I realized how emotionally abusive my parents had been. Bob had protected me from them. After he died, they again began treating me as they had when I was a child. After being in a relationship for twenty years, surrounded by unconditional love, where I had been adored and valued, I realized I deserved more than what I had endured while growing up.

When my mother fell in the library room, spraining her wrist and breaking her finger, she blamed it on a desk drawer that had been partially left open, causing her to trip. When she fell walking to the car, the uneven bricks in the pathway were at fault for her tumble. After a few more meetings of ground and flesh, a visit to the doctor and a battery of specialized tests were in order.

In 2006, the person who, for over forty years, had allowed nothing to pass her lips that was not organic, sugar-free, whole wheat, containing no preservatives or additives, who had exercised daily for over four decades, was diagnosed with Lou Gehrig's disease.

Lou Gehrig's disease, or ALS, is a cruel and devastating diagnosis and illness. I had never known anyone with Lou Gehrig's disease and was naïve as to the progression of this debilitating and ultimately fatal disease. How someone, who had taken for so many years the best care of her physical needs of anyone I have ever known, could develop an illness that would rob her body of all functions was unfathomable.

The progression was incremental and linear, and over time, it gained full control over my mother's body—one muscle, one joint, and one organ at a time. Following her rapid succession of falls, my mother began using a walking stick for support and stability. The stick was tall, gnarled, and brightly painted with an African motif. In the beginning of her illness, that stick was never far from her side. Soon, a mechanical chair lift was installed to elevate her from the first floor to the upstairs bedroom.

When the stick no longer offered security from falling, my mother transitioned to a walker. She was always fiercely independent, and when the walker failed and a wheelchair became necessary, it was motorized so that she could drive herself. That wheelchair became a menace as my mother's muscular prowess deteriorated, and she ran into cupboards, the refrigerator, door frames, and furniture. But there was no convincing my mother to give up the last vestiges of her independence.

Until she had to. The progression of the disease atrophied all her muscles, and when she was unable to hold her torso erect, she was relegated to laying down. A hospital bed was installed next to the mahogany bed from her trousseau sixty years prior. With my father sleeping alone in the antique bed, my mother could be raised to a sitting position with the help of the hospital bed hydraulics. Meals were transported upstairs via the stair chair, and her bedroom became the living—and dying—room of the house.

With catheters installed and stomach tubes surgically implanted, hospice services were engaged. Although the muscles required for speech had deteriorated, my mother never lost her voice. She scratched notes nearly unintelligible for most, but my educator-trained eye could decipher the scribbles. Through these directives, my mother made her wishes known.

Although past emotional wounds made it painful to do, I took care of my mother as the slippery slope of ALS dragged her down its abyss. Visiting and feeding her daily, interpreting her notes, and ensuring all her wishes were met by her caregivers was made possible only by choking down and compartmentalizing my rage from her neglect and disdain of me for half a century.

Each time I left my mother's bedside, I said, "I love you," sending those words across the medicinal air. I hoped my words would inspire a reciprocal sentiment but my endearments always fell flat, landing with a thud on non-deaf ears, a sense surprisingly unimpaired by this insidious disease.

Once my mother became unable to swallow solid food, I spoon-fed her cracked ice with a little juice mixed in. Now unable to put pen to paper, she struggled to get words out to issue her directives. One day, garbled sounds strung together with frantic ferocity as my mother forced out, "I mo ju."

Nearly dropping the spoon and cracked ice, I twisted my head toward my mother.

Hoping beyond hope, I asked softly, "Did you say 'I love you?'"

Clenching her eyes, head wagging back and forth on her pillow, she stated more emphatically, "Mo ju."

Then I understood.

"Oh. You meant more juice."

Descending the stairs to the kitchen, I chastised myself for my weakness and stupidity. Now fifty-seven, the little girl in me had still hoped my mother was finally telling me she loved me—for the first time in my entire life.

Unlike my father, whose mental decline became more pronounced when he turned ninety, my mother never lost one iota of mental acuity. She remained true to herself and her convictions until the day the involuntary muscles of her lungs lost the ability to expand and contract. When her last breath was taken, with it went her resolve to ensure I would never know what it would be like to be told I was loved by my mother.

When the Shomer and chevra kadisha came to bathe and wrap my mother in white linen to carry her away, her limp, lifeless, and now feather-light body was jostled while maneuvered into the white cocoon body bag. I implored them to be more careful and respectful. My mother's struggles were over. Mine would continue to haunt me.

I do not miss my mother or father, who died eleven years after my mother.

What I miss is the opportunity to know what it might have been like to grow up—and be grown up—in a family where I was wanted, cherished, and loved. Despite the pain and damage my mother inflicted upon me for more than half my life, I need never feel guilt or regret. I didn't abandon my mother throughout her illness and journey toward death; for me that option was never a possibility. I had been well trained by my parents to "make nice," trying to be accepted and loved by them. Although my efforts to please never accomplished that, those skills served me well as I cared for my mother when she needed it most.

Standing on the deck of the house she would soon purchase with her late husband, Bob, a black and white dairy cow stood on the hillside. Growing up on Long Island and never having been around cows, Janet proclaimed this was no place to raise children. Now nearly five decades later, Janet is a full-time farmer with a herd of seventy long-haired, long-horned Highland cows. Prior to raising cattle Janet taught first grade for thirty years and was named Vermont Teacher of the Year in 2002. Janet's photojournalism has been published in *Vermont Life*, *American Forests Magazine*, *Yankee Magazine*, and the *Heartland Highland Journal*. Janet believes writing enabled her to get through the grief of losing Bob and the pain of her challenging childhood.

OF YEARS OF LOVE, AND A LONG GOODBYE BOB COUSY

by Dianne Williamson

The following first appeared in the Worcester TELEGRAM & GAZETTE on September 29, 2013. Printed with permission from the publisher. Dianne Williamson was the columnist who wrote the story.

The game plan, as he called it, rarely varied. Each morning, he'd awaken first and set things on the kitchen table — her pills, the newspaper, a fiber bar, a banana. Then he'd return to the bedroom and rouse his wife. Often, she balked at leaving the warmth of the covers, so he'd gently coax her. Always, he was gentle.

Once she was up, he'd lead her to the kitchen to read the newspaper. It took two or three hours to get through the pages, because she'd underline each sentence in every story with a black pen. After a while he found comfort in reading between the lines, because it was something they shared.

""She was leading a happy life," he said. "It was part of the game plan."

Bob Cousy knows a bit about game plans, and he and his wife, Missie, were always a team. In the early days of their marriage, when the Celtics star was gone for weeks at a time, Missie made her husband a presence in the family home by telling her daughters where he was and what he was doing. Decades later, when Missie slowly succumbed to the ravages of dementia, her husband ensured that the woman he called "my bride" was always by his side, even as her mind wandered where he couldn't follow.

Last week, after 63 years of marriage, Bob Cousy said goodbye to his bride. His loved ones say he's bereft, inconsolable. And they're surprised that he agreed to an interview, because Cousy is a private man who cared for Missie alone for more than a decade, never seeking help, services or sympathy. That wasn't in the game plan.

Cousy married his high school sweetheart, the raven-haired Marie Ritterbusch, six months after he graduated from the College of the Holy Cross, where he helped his team win an NCAA championship in 1947. He spent his wedding night playing point guard for the Celtics. Days later, he left for a two-week road trip.

The grueling travel schedule would define the first half of their marriage. While her husband was transforming the game of basketball and later worked as a coach and sports commentator, Missie raised two daughters and instilled in them her passion for civil rights and the peace movement. Quick-witted, beautiful and kind, she was a mentor to the new Celtics' wives and especially embraced the wives of black players such as Bill Russell and Jo Jo White. She was a Girl Scout leader and a gardener, a fiercely independent woman who could discuss politics with the same skill she applied to the faulty plumbing in the family's English Tudor on Salisbury Street.

"I was busy playing a child's game," Cousy said last week, sitting in the living room with daughters Marie and Ticia. "I thought putting a ball in a hole was important. Looking back, I should have participated more in the lives of my family. But my girls were in the best possible loving hands."

Today, the Celtic legend known as "Cooz" is 85 but looks younger by a decade. Articulate and gracious, he tears up easily when discussing his wife and the love affair that flourished as the couple aged.

"Our marriage was somewhat contrary to tradition," he said. "Most couples have the most intensity in the beginning. But I was always working. So we had the best and most romantic part of our marriage at the end. We literally held hands for the last 20 years."

Missie's cognitive decline was gradual and began a dozen years ago, Cousy said. She would ask him the same question, over and over. She hallucinated, grew disoriented and struggled with balance. But she always knew her husband, and she bristled at any suggestion that she suffered from dementia.

So Cousy worked hard to create the perception that his once-independent wife was vital and healthy. Because she believed she could still drive, he shipped her station wagon to their place in Florida each winter so she could see it in the driveway. Artificial red flowers were planted in her garden. He did all the household chores and let her think she performed them herself.

"My dad provided an environment that allowed her, in her mind, to be a fully functioning adult," said daughter Marie. "It was amazing to watch."

The couple's social life vanished as Missie's symptoms worsened. Other than a Thursday night "out with the boys" and some quick rounds of golf, Cousy spent all of his time alone with his bride. He watched "General Hospital" with Missie and patiently answered the same questions. He stocked the fridge with her favorite candy, Reese's Peanut Butter Cups. At night, she'd cover him with a blanket and he'd stroke her arm.

"I love you, honey," he'd say.

"I love you, too," Missie would always reply.

The sports legend who led the Celtics to six World Championships said he never felt defeated by the challenge of caring full-time for his ailing spouse.

"It drew us closer together," he said. "It was never a chore, because I knew she would have done the same for me. You just have to go with the flow. Every three months, I'd scream out something just for release."

On Sept. 7, Cousy took his wife for an early dinner at Worcester Country Club. On the way home, in the car, Missie suffered a massive stroke. She died peacefully two weeks later and was buried in St. John's Cemetery.

WARM, PEACEFUL, AND COZY

by Sarah Britton

with Mark J. Resnick

Prostate cancer is one of the most curable cancers—if caught early. To catch it, you simply need your doctor to authorize a Prostate-specific antigen test (PSA), which measures the level of PSA in the blood. Measured in nanograms per milliliter (ng/md) of blood, the normal range is in the low single digits. By the time my father had his PSA test, it was too late.

Mom and Dad retired to Zirconia, North Carolina, and were very happy there. Each time I asked them to consider moving back to Vermont to be closer to me, they scoffed at the idea.

In 2018, something unexpected happened—something big—I got pregnant at age forty. My sister and her husband decided against having children, so I was my parents' only hope of having grandchildren. The only trouble was, my partner and I had been trying for nearly a year with no success. Mom and Dad had given up any hope of being grandparents, but when they got the call from me about my pregnancy, they were cautiously excited. Seeing the baby's face on the ultrasound made it real—for all of us.

"Come up and be grandparents," I pitched the idea again. "I know it's cold, but it'll be fun."

They agreed. Without protest or uncertainty, they said yes. My dad visited, bought a house, and began packing up the van, but not before he said he would need to see a doctor when he arrived. That was odd, as my dad never went to see a doctor. Something must be up. Why would he so readily agree to move up here, and then insist on seeing a doctor?

I was a nurse practitioner for a busy orthopedic practice in Vermont. I called in a few favors to get him an appointment the following week. It was no easy task to arrange this, and I'm so thankful for knowing how to navigate the healthcare system. I can't imagine how people without inside help manage to get the care they need.

Days later, Mom and Dad arrived and began unpacking their stuff. I knew my dad was experiencing some back pain but still didn't know what the issue was. We found out rather quickly at his appointment. The doctor tested his blood, and the results were shocking: his PSA was 312. The follow-up CT scan confirmed he had cancer; worse, it had metastasized, invading his ureters and kidneys. The joy of having my parents move back to Vermont had taken an unexpected and desperate turn, all within a matter of days.

My caregiving duties began immediately. His medical team installed nephrostomy tubes, which helped manage Dad's pain. The tubes were in for six months, then stents were put in place to open the tubes from the ureter to the bladder. The tubes required a lot of maintenance. Not only did we have to change the dressings where the tubes were inserted, but we had to flush the tubes with syringes every day. Sometimes they would leak or get crusty. I taught my mom how to clean them, and it was a stressful job for us both.

Managing his medicines was my job, as were his doctors' appointments. Again, I kept asking myself, *How do people do this if they're not in health care?* The burden the system puts on unpaid and untrained family members is astounding. It was tough for me, and I knew how to navigate the system.

Every time my phone rang, I thought, *Oh no, what happened or what's wrong now?* To make matters worse, the chemotherapy wasn't working. While waiting for an appointment at Dana Farber to discuss a new treatment plan, we met with palliative care. It wasn't his idea; I set it up. Dad and I never spoke bluntly about his cancer or treatment plan. The research shows that a positive outlook can give a patient more time. It's not that he wasn't positive, but as it turned out, he knew all of what we were hiding, especially that his chances of surviving his cancer were 2%

I was direct with him anyway.

"If the experimental drug treatment at Dana Farber doesn't work, there aren't any other treatment options."

"Sarah, I know. I'm well aware my life expectancy is five years."

"Can I do something? Should we make plans?"

Per his wishes, there would be no funeral, and he would be cremated. After making his intentions known, he shared the story about when his tonsils were removed when he was a boy. When he went under during anesthesia, he remembers seeing himself on the table—the doctors and nurses were working on him. "It was an unbelievably good feeling. Warm, peaceful, and cozy." He never told me that story before.

Every three months, Dad had to get the stents taken out and replaced. The cancerous tissue took over his body. For the last year, year and half, the tubes went back in, complete with urine bags on the outside. Near the end, while trying to procure a urine sample for the doctor, he couldn't do it. He couldn't get his pants on or off anymore.

Still, his passing was unexpectedly unexpected. We knew he was going to die from prostate cancer. He had five years to live, at most, and he was in year four. I thought we had a little more time, but it wasn't part of his plan.

The night he died, he sat up in bed and announced, "It's time to go." Then my mom said he just collapsed on the bed. My mom asked him, ""Do you mean it's time to die?"

He nodded.

Then she asked, "Do you want me to call an ambulance?"

He nodded.

When I got to the hospital, he was hooked up to monitors and machines. He looked terrible. The beeping of the machines agitated him, and he kept pulling at my hand. I just knew this was it.

"Are you in pain?"

Again, he nodded.

Just as the doctor came into the room, I told the nurse he needed pain medication through his IV. The nurse had been holding off on providing it because the medicine tanks your vitals. In his case, it would be helping him die. She held firm.

"Do you want us to be aggressive to save you?" I asked Dad.

He shook his head no, so I again asked for the pain medication.

"Why don't you ask the family, who is standing in front of you, what he wants," I said to the nurse.

Finally, the doctor agreed, but Dad still kept tugging at my hand.

"What's wrong. Is it the beeping?"

He nodded yes.

"Please turn it all off. All the machines."

My sister had come in from Tennessee and was staying with us, but when we called the ambulance, she was already asleep, as was my son. We didn't want him seeing them take his Pop Pop away in an ambulance. So it was just me and my mom.

I remember him telling me, "I'm not afraid to die. I know I'm going to feel good—peaceful—just like when I had the tonsils out."

The machines no longer beeped, and the room was quiet. I don't know if it was a smile on his face, but when he took his last breath, I knew he was finally at peace.

It's sad that many of us don't have these relationships with our parents until they reach retirement age or get sick. Had my parents not moved up to Vermont, I'm not sure how they would have managed. When I first got pregnant, they said "No thanks," but my mom felt like it was a divine intervention. Something in the cosmos brought them to Vermont as if someone knew. I'm thankful for the time with him; it was the most meaningful years we had together.

My son still talks about his Pop Pop, and Dad got to see his second grandson before he died. I always feel like he's here, somewhere. Mom says the same thing. One time she was in our living room, and all the lights went off in the house. Then they came back. "That was Dad," she said.

That same week, I woke up in the middle of the night and swore I heard a man urinating in our bathroom. I didn't know what was happening, but I just lay there. Then the sound went away. Was that my dad telling me that his pipes were working now because that's something he would have done. *He was ever the prankster.*

There was a time after his diagnosis in which I was very angry with my dad for not going to the doctor. When he was living in North Carolina, I reminded him often to get his blood work and screening done.

"Yeah, I'm going to do that."

I was even angrier at myself for not making him go.

Watching him decline was hard and stressful. He was always the strong one and very independent. He changed the oil in the cars, fixed the lawnmowers, and stacked the wood. We had three good years and only one bad with him in Vermont. His mind stayed sharp until the end, so we were lucky in that regard.

I was very sad when he passed away. We were close. But at the same time, there was a huge sense of relief. When I think about him, I don't see him as sick or weak or fragile. I think of him in Heaven as happy and strong, playing music and hanging with his dog, Buster.

How could I be sad, knowing that he's warm, peaceful, and cozy again?

THRIVING WITH ASPERGER'S SYNDROME

by Jennifer Osborne

My son Doug is a handsome, athletic, and intelligent forty-one-year-old man. Looking at him, one might never imagine the hurdles he has faced to get to this point in his life.

He owns and maintains a beautiful house. He is an accomplished software developer, writer, and athlete. He is a loving son, nephew, and friend, as well as a devoted "dad" to his sweet dachshund, Jessie.

It was not always this way.

Doug has autism spectrum disorder (Asperger's syndrome) and ADHD. At times, he has also suffered from severe depression and anxiety. All of these have caused many struggles in his young life. It is nothing short of miraculous that he has gotten to the place he is now.

As his mother, I have been the primary overseer of his care and, much of the time, his only support system. His beloved older brother died tragically when Doug was just fourteen and had just begun high school. This left him without the one person I always knew would be his greatest friend and supporter in life.

Many times, I didn't think I could do what was necessary to help Doug fight his demons. I have had to intervene when I thought he may be dead, to learn to offer support instead of criticism, and perhaps hardest of all, to hold my tongue even when he was clearly self-destructive.

There were times I wanted to pack a bag and run away. Some people in my orbit suggested that I do just that, although I no longer consider them to be my "friends." I knew my heart would never allow me to abandon Doug. I knew that no matter what, I would always fight alongside him so he could conquer his challenges and lead the life he deserves.

Doug wasn't diagnosed with Asperger's until he was twenty-two. As a child, he was exceptionally bright, happy, and playful. He excelled at school and in sports.

There were subtle signs of Doug's Asperger's from a young age, although autism was very rarely diagnosed back in the 1980s. His speech development was slightly delayed, and he didn't start to talk until after his second birthday. His kindergarten teacher was concerned about his speech and consulted the school therapist, but the therapist determined there was nothing wrong with him or his speech. He just preferred not to speak much and instead would play math games and even chess with his friends. I always attributed it to the fact that his older brother was extremely outgoing and precocious in his communication skills. His brother spoke for him, I told myself, though Doug was hardly a mute.

While his brother excelled verbally, Doug was a math prodigy in high school. As an accomplished "mathlete" and captain of his high school math team, he received numerous awards and a perfect score on his math SAT. Hardly a child who showed signs of any problems except perhaps his unusual abilities. Doug was far from perfect in high school, but his high school years began about as far from perfect as possible.

Fast forward to when I first became aware of the signs of Doug's autism and how it had caused him difficulties. I was filled with guilt for not recognizing his distinctive qualities as unusual. I tried to play "catch up" by getting him all the help I could. I leaned on my own therapist to forgive myself for failing the child I loved so much. I learned to substitute my own self-destructive habits with healthier ways (for both of us) to deal with my Pandora's box of emotions. And I learned how to hold on for survival, his and mine, as we rode this rollercoaster that daily life became.

In spite, or perhaps because of his Asperger's, Doug managed to build a successful career as a software engineer in his twenties and early thirties. He was at his best between 2009 and 2013 when he was working from his home in Connecticut, and I was living just three miles down the road.

Doug's unusual way of thinking due to his autism has been an equal contributor to his successes and his failures. At the end of 2013, his successes led to him accepting a senior software engineer position at a top tech company in Chicago. His move to Chicago was the catalyst of a downward spiral that took years to fully recover from.

Doug's darkest hours occurred at the beginning of 2016 when he was still living in Chicago but was no longer employed. Doug had isolated himself from the world and was completely out of touch. I was so worried that I would call his apartment complex just to make sure he was still alive. In March, I received a call from his best friend, who thought I should fly out to Chicago to bring Doug back to Connecticut. The next day, I was in Chicago, and I brought Doug home the following day.

The next few years were very difficult for both of us, as Doug was suffering from anxiety and severe depression. I had to learn how to separate Doug, my son, from the at-times hurtful person who seemed to know just how to stab my gut and make me crumble in pain. It was not Doug behaving this way; it was his illness.

But it was hard. *So hard.* Besides my therapist, there were few people I felt I could share my struggles with. In my family, all the bad parts in life were swept under the carpet. I had been taught not to discuss this nightmare we were living. When I tried to be open about it, even my close friends became tired of hearing about my pain. Many couldn't understand Doug's illness and often referred to his problems as "issues," a term I've always objected to. Show me a person without "issues," and I will show you a person who is in denial or self-medicating in some way.

Eventually, I rarely spoke of the reality of my life. As a professional opera singer and voice teacher, I tried to focus on my music and bury my emotional pain. I couldn't learn enough new music and vocal pedagogy. There was only one person I ever shared my problems with: Evelyn, my beloved voice teacher and friend. Without Evelyn pushing me to not only keep going but to find a source of joy in my life again, I am not even sure that I would be here now.

They say that having a child is like having your heart outside of your own body. How true this is. I couldn't imagine having any peace in life while Doug was struggling, and I still can't. My heart has been battered and beaten to a pulp. Through no fault of his own, but because of Doug's autism and temporary illness that have made his life complicated and challenging. Whatever pain I have felt, his has been tenfold.

It has been a long journey, but Doug has overcome his challenges and emerged on the other side. I like to think that my support helped him get there, but mostly, it was his work and unfailing persistence. Doug's perseverance has become an inspiration to others experiencing life's challenges, both on and off the autism spectrum.

I can't change the past or predict the future. But I can promise that whatever transpires, my son can and will survive and, more than that, thrive.

And I wouldn't exchange being Doug's mother, through good times and bad, for all the riches in the world.

SHE'S JUST LIKE YOU

by Fredda Fox Stimell

with Mark J. Resnick

My older brother had mental health issues, and it was hard on the whole family to see him suffer for so many years. You never forget it—watching someone go through the pain of depression and other mood disorders. When it was time to consider having children of my own, it was always on my mind. I didn't want to bring a child into this world who might suffer the same fate as my brother, though I never expressed this fear with anyone, including my husband.

I pushed those thoughts aside during my first two pregnancies and was blessed with two beautiful children, a girl and a boy. When my husband Herbie and I decided to have one more baby, I would be lying if I didn't admit to myself, *Maybe I am pushing my luck.*

I was thirty-two when my third child, Nancy, was born. Nancy was born at Mount Sinai Hospital in New York City. Even though we lived on Long Island, we drove into the city each time so I could be with the same doctor.

It was a normal delivery, but my husband told me that Nancy had problems, and the doctors didn't want me to see her yet. Then, I was told that she was a dying baby, and I panicked. I got a hold of a nurse and demanded to see Nancy, who was in the intensive care unit. If I hadn't insisted, they wouldn't have let me see her.

There she was, kicking, but all hooked up to tubes. I thought, *That's not my baby who is dying; that's a baby fighting for her life.* It was apparent to me, however, that nobody wanted me to get too attached to her. I know that sounds awful, but back then, it wasn't a given that parents kept babies who had problems based on little or inaccurate information from medical personnel. Many parents put their infants who were developmentally delayed into private institutions, which was what my husband and I did.

We visited Nancy in upstate New York and took our children with us each time. One of my aunts and my mother offered to take her to Florida to care for her full-time, but I couldn't do that. How could I explain to my children that my mother and aunt could take care of her but I could not?

Shortly after, we took her out of the institution. Our next best option was to get her placed in foster care, which was where Nancy stayed in a community not far from us on Long Island, where we continued to visit her often with the children. She lived with her foster family from the age of three months until her second birthday.

Then came the life-changing phone call. The social worker assigned to Nancy's case called and gave me an ultimatum: take her home or give her up for adoption. I immediately called my husband at work.

"What are we going to do?" I asked.

"It's your call, Fredda. You're going to be the primary caregiver for her. I'll be working, so the burden will fall on you."

"That's not fair, Herbie. We need to make this decision together."

My oldest daughter, Mindy, was five, and her brother, Scott, was three. Mindy wanted that baby home.

"Why isn't she home?" she asked.

I had to run through a list of reasons, including the fact that she may never be able to walk or talk. I was most afraid that having Nancy with us would negatively impact Mindy and Scott's childhood and happiness. Again, I know I sound like a monster but these were, unfortunately, common opinions in the late 1960s.

Mindy never relented. "I don't care—I want my sister!" And she was right. Nancy belonged with us. If the foster family could care for her, then why couldn't we? As a family, we decided to take her back home with us. If Herbie and I couldn't make it work, for whatever reason, we knew we could put her up for adoption.

The day we took Nancy home from foster care, however, she was a very sad little girl. She was happy with her foster care home. They were the only family she knew. Oh, how hard it must have been for her to understand why she had to leave them.

Right away, Scott and Mindy loved Nancy—it was as if she was always with us. Scott made her laugh nonstop. He would run around the house and do silly things to make her laugh and feel comfortable. Mindy got to her through music, playing the piano, and singing. I, on the other hand, was struggling.

It took me a while for me to love her with the same depth as my first two children. I thought people looked at me in the supermarket because Nancy looked different. Her physical milestones were also very delayed. Mostly, I was petrified that people wouldn't accept her or that Mindy and Scott's friends would treat them differently once they saw Nancy.

My fears were unwarranted. Everyone who met Nancy was warm and welcoming. Neighbors, friends, other family members—everyone. Around this time, I became involved in the Down syndrome community, which forever changed my life. I became a positive force and leader within the community. I wasn't just an advocate for Nancy, but for all the children. My husband was too. We were a great team.

What most people don't realize is that children with Down syndrome are more like other children than they are different. They have the same feelings as other children—they cry; they need to go the bathroom at the most inopportune times; they get angry, sick, and insulted. Just like every other child. Each child born with Down syndrome has their own personality. People assume that they are always happy and smiley, but their moods are no different than anyone else's. More importantly, they understand right from wrong.

Nancy's vocabulary was her strong point. She would say to me, "That's not appropriate, Mom." I spent a lot of time reading her poetry and playing rhyme games—just like I did with Mindy and Scott. The way she sounded was different, but she still had the innate knowledge and skills to play little league, attend plays and concerts, and take piano and typing lessons. All of these activities gave her critical lifelong skills to communicate and assimilate to most situations.

The hardest aspect of having a child with Down syndrome or special needs is the fear that their health will fail. Nancy didn't have any heart issues or hearing loss, which is common for people with Down syndrome, but I was worried that I would have to take care of her the rest of my life, physically and financially. Herbie and I declared her incompetent with the New York State courts to ensure she would get the services in which she was entitled. Unfortunately, at that time, you didn't automatically get them.

I was also afraid that kids would pick on Nancy—or that Mindy and Scott would resent us for taking time away from them to care for her. Again, my fears were completely unwarranted. Nancy was an absolute asset to our family. She was kind, caring, socially smart, and so full of love. Our lives changed completely from the moment we brought her home—and for the better. As a matter of fact, for the important milestones in Nancy's life, Mindy and Scott's friends asked to be invited.

It wasn't just Herbie and I who fully immersed ourselves in the Down syndrome community. Mindy and Scott were very much a part of everything. As a family, we helped a lot of people. Strangers sometimes showed up unannounced in my backyard during the weekend, holding a baby with Down syndrome. We did whatever we could to support and encourage those complete strangers. It took some time, but I realized that this was my calling in life.

Maria and Bill Hartman sought and received approval from the State of New York to create a nonprofit organization called the Association for Children with Down Syndrome. There was very little research on Down syndrome, and almost all the information was negative. We not only helped the Hartmans but also worked with a group of parents who ran an informal preschool for children with Down syndrome.

All of us were unpaid volunteers. There was no funding whatsoever at this point, but the school got a major boost after Herbie and I formed a relationship with North Shore University Hospital's Child Development Center. Through a letter and handshake, we worked with Dr. Jessica Davis and her professional medical team, who provided guidance and support to our staff. This relationship proved to be instrumental in the school's growth.

In order to expand and validate the preschool, we went to the Bellmore School District and presented a plan to have our program housed in a public-school classroom. This was unheard of at the time—a private non-profit using a public school facility. They agreed, in large part because they saw we had the support of Dr. Davis and her team.

The next logical step was to get certification and funding for a New York State Family Courts Early Intervention Program, which we did. But we didn't stop there. Next, we got them to fund a bus for children to attend the preschool. That's right, transportation was provided for infants with Down syndrome to get to school.

Herbie and I spoke as often as we could to groups about Down syndrome. Here's what I would say to the classroom, whether they had Down syndrome or not.

"Is the person next to you doing anything differently than you? Maybe they sound different, but he or she says the same things you do. Can you tell me what their IQ is? Do you even care what his IQ is? No. What do you care about? That he is nice and can play with you."

And to the older kids, I would bring up Einstein's theory of relativity by saying, "I know about Einstein's theory, but I don't understand it. And I don't really care to understand it. Does anybody in this room care if I understand it? As long as I know the basics of what it is, we can have a conversation. The same holds true for persons with Down syndrome. They need to become aware of what's going on in society to be participating members—and to be someone's friend."

I never considered myself a caregiver for Nancy. She was my child, and I was her mom. I took care of her the same way I took care of Mindy and Scott. Nancy has been the major ingredient in making my family special. I consider myself very lucky to have her. What I thought was a burden became a blessing.

Fredda Fox Stimell is a retired Executive Director of the Association for Children with Down Syndrome (ACDS) on Long Island, NY. She was married to the late Herbert Stimell and has three adult children. She currently resides in New York City.

HOW CANCER WILL CHANGE YOUR LIFE

by Michael D. Tenaglia

In early February 2013, my family and I were celebrating two birthdays, including mine and my mother-in-law, who was about to reach the young age of ninety. We shared cake, ice cream, and drinks but were also mindful that my wife, Lynda, was days from having a tumor near her thyroid removed.

It was a five-centimeter tumor, but all indications were that it was benign, and she had one of the best local surgeons performing the operation. Once the tumor was removed, she would be fine in a few days. Cancer was the furthest thing on her mind, especially since her most recent visit with her internist showed that everything was fine. Only it wasn't.

Lynda began to notice that her voice was "not quite normal" and that she could not project it the same way as in the past. Her doctor referred her to Massachusetts General Hospital's Voice Center to determine the condition of her vocal cords. Outwardly, the MGH Voice Center is a medical facility. But when you look more closely at the walls, photos, and messages of appreciation from celebrities, you realize that you are in one of the finest institutions in the world. I felt so fortunate to have this facility twenty minutes from my home, especially knowing that others come from all over the world for treatment.

Unfortunately, further testing confirmed the presence of the tumor and that one of her vocal cords was "frozen;" it did not move, which meant that her voice relied on a particular cord closest to the tumor. Still, there was no indication that the cancer was malignant. A biopsy was impossible because the tumor was too big, so the recommendation was to have surgery to remove it.

Cancer can strike at any time, but to everyone else—definitely not you or someone close to you. When you suspect something is wrong, it's too common to go about your daily business. That's where my head was, anyway.

Doctors give you hope and assurance that everything will be okay. Looking back, I was in denial. Even though I had lost my father and uncle to cancer, I was optimistic for Lynda. Or maybe my head was just in the sand. You always hope for the best—isn't that what keeps us going?

The day before Lynda's surgery, I went to work with my usual energy, enthusiasm, and expectations for a Monday. I made my regular stop at Dunkin Donuts in Concord, MA, and I arrived at my office at the usual time of 6:45 a.m. I wanted to finish a few things and meet with my staff because I would be out the rest of the week taking care of Lynda.

I met with my boss and asked if he wanted me to work on anything special. "Just take care of your wife," he said, which I appreciated. Even still, I said that she would be resting and would have nothing to do, so I wanted to work on something. As usual, I brought work home, fully expecting I could get things done on my laptop or phone.

Lynda and I stuck to our regular morning routines on the day of her surgery. There was the usual light talk while we waited for her to enter the operating room. Once again, the doctor reassured us that everything would be fine. She told me to go home and wait for the call, which would be in two to three hours. So I went home and walked Sophie, our dog, and waited.

She went into surgery at 8:00 a.m. I expected the call to come at the earliest proposed time (10:00 a.m.). I remember sitting on the couch with Sophie, waiting for the phone to ring. At 10:30 a.m., I started to get a little nervous. At 11:00 a.m., I called the hospital to see what was happening and was told they were still in surgery. I still thought that everything would be okay.

I didn't know that the rest of our lives would change.

The doctor called me slightly after 12:00 p.m., four hours after Lynda entered the Operating Room. *What took so long?* Dr. Stephen explained that they found cancer and called in some specialists to confirm. They could not remove the entire tumor, nor the thyroid, because it was wrapped around the vocal cord. They decided not to remove it all because of the high probability that the one remaining vocal cord would be damaged and she would lose her ability to speak.

My mind went blank as Dr. Stephen spoke with me, explaining the surgery and what she had done. I didn't hear anything after the words *cancer* and *malignant*. I only thought of Lynda and what I had to do to support her. I also thought about our daughter, Maria, and how I would tell her the terrible news and support her simultaneously.

I thought I would have at least a few moments to gather my thoughts before telling Maria the awful news—to try and put some positive spin on what I had just learned. I didn't get the chance to gather my thoughts because, as I was speaking with Dr. Stephen, my cell phone rang. It was Maria. I had to answer. What would she think if I did not answer?

I switched to my cell phone and broke down on the phone with Maria. I told her that it was cancer, and tears flowed.

I regret not being able to shield my daughter from this terrible news and that I could no longer speak after the word "cancer." I don't know where Maria was when we spoke, but she was at my house ten minutes later. We called Dr. Stephen back and asked if we could meet with her that afternoon to learn more and decide how we would break the news to Lynda. We cried and told each other we had to be strong for Mom.

Dr. Stephen was extremely patient and explained that this was papillary thyroid cancer and that it was treatable. Lynda could live a long life with treatment. I was relieved; at the time, I did not understand the difference between treatment and cure. She also mentioned that the pathology report was not yet in, and we did not know the full extent of her cancer.

Dr. Stephen agreed that she should be the one to speak with Lynda, tell her the diagnosis, and explain the next steps to bring her back to good health.

That night, we visited with Lynda in her room. It was a challenging conversation because Maria and I knew the outcome, but the meeting between Lynda and Dr. Stephen wasn't until the following day. We had to maintain a positive tone and give Lynda an optimistic outlook—all the while knowing that she had been cursed with a malignant cancerous tumor.

I went home and tried to get some rest, but it was pointless. Who could sleep after what had just transpired earlier that day? My mind wandered to what we were about to go through and how we could provide comfort and support to Lynda.

As agreed, Maria and I met with Dr. Stephen the following morning, and the three of us walked into Lynda's room. She was in good spirits. Dr. Stephen explained the procedure and told Lynda that they found a malignant cancerous tumor, a treatable form of papillary thyroid cancer. I watched Lynda's face as she heard the news and saw that it took her breath away.

It was a good and appropriate time to interject humor into the conversation. Maria chimed in by saying, "Don't worry, Ma, you will die from living with Dad rather than this cancer." Dr. Stephen then recommended that we schedule an appointment with Dr. Lori Wirth at Massachusetts General Hospital. A referral for which we are very grateful, even to this day.

We met with Dr. Wirth and her team two weeks later. They took time to explain the disease and the process of chemotherapy and radiation. They also had words of encouragement for Lynda. Some doctors showed more compassion than others, but I was confident they could see Lynda through the next seven weeks of chemotherapy and radiation. At this point, the focus was on Lynda and treating the disease. I felt good about my role as a caregiver.

We all know someone who has been touched by cancer. I lost my father to cancer in 1971 and an uncle in 1996. I was twenty-three years old and just married when my father was diagnosed, but I did not understand his cancer's full impact because my mother was his primary caregiver. I didn't fully understand the effect his cancer had on our family.

Throughout Dad's cancer battle, I was shielded by my mother and by the fact that I was not living at home and seeing every minute of what cancer does to a person. I wish I had known what my mother went through. I still regret my failure to support her as a son—to be there for her. At the time, I thought I was doing it all, as I had started a new job and had my own new family.

I know now that it was not enough.

Caring for a person living in the same house is an entirely different experience. Still, I was comforted knowing that Lynda had the best medical care in the world just minutes from our home. I tend to be optimistic and always think things will be okay, which is the right attitude.

Be positive in your outlook, but don't lose sight of the fact that you are dealing with a challenging disease that can devastate you and your family. The stress of caregiving can cause more illnesses, so find a way to stay focused yet positive. And make time to relieve some of the accumulated stress that inevitably comes with caring for a loved one with cancer.

Our daily visits to Mass General started with radiation at 8:00 a.m. On Wednesdays, she would have a blood test and chemotherapy, which would last up to six hours. I spoke with my boss about the schedule and asked for the flexibility to come in after radiation, which he approved. On some days, Maria would take her to Mass General so I could be at work at my normal 7:00 a.m. time. I was blessed to have worked for a great company, and they supported me every step.

I can do this.

During one radiation visit, a nurse met with us and asked how I was doing. I explained that I was doing fine and receiving help from our daughter, Maria. But the truth was, between work and caring for Lynda, I was not okay. It was beginning to take a toll on my mental and physical health. In my mind, I was strong, in good health, and could work endless hours at home or the office to make up for the days when I would be late.

The nurse suggested that I consider taking a leave of absence. I said no, I work for a company that understands my situation, so it would not be necessary. I thought the idea of taking a leave of absence was nonsense. I considered it a personal failure if I couldn't do this, especially with help from Maria. Together, we would see Lynda through this, so we stayed on this schedule for three weeks.

I could not have been more wrong.

While Lynda was getting the physical treatment for cancer, I forgot the emotional and mental impact that cancer has on a person. She was alone most of the day, and when one is alone, the mind wonders and conjures all sorts of worrisome and stressful scenarios.

I was also paying the price of splitting my time between home and work. My mind wandered to Lynda when I was in the office, and when I was home with Lynda, my mind wandered to the work piling up at the office. I finally realized that I was not being effective in either role as husband and caregiver or as senior vice president of a bank.

When Lynda's medical team wanted to have a feeding tube placed inside Lynda's throat because of the swelling from the radiation, and I saw her anguishing every minute of the day, I knew it was time to step away from work. I witnessed the side effects of her treatment wreak havoc on her mind and body. The same blistering radiation burn noticeable on the outside of her neck was also on the inside, only it wasn't evident to us.

Lynda was strong and persevered through it all. She later said she had to be strong for the rest of us.

Many nights, Lynda was sick from the chemotherapy, and neither one of us could get any sleep. There were nights when we had to go to Mass General for medication to counter the effects of chemotherapy. We would be up until the early morning hours and then had to get up for radiation, chemotherapy, and work.

People would often ask about Lynda, but rarely did anyone ask how Maria and I were doing. If asked, I would tell them we were doing fine, but it wasn't true. Consciously, I believed that we were doing fine, but it was taking its toll, and concentrating on anything except Lynda was getting harder. Where can you go for help?

As a side note, Lynda's daily visits to Mass General in April **2013** coincided with the Boston Marathon. We made our daily visit to Mass General for radiation, went home, and then I returned to my office. At 2:49 p.m., the bomb went off, and news traveled fast. At approximately 3:00 p.m., my office went silent because of the bomb at the finish line. I thought of Lynda and a friend whose daughter was running the Marathon. I called Lynda to see how she was doing and then called my friend at the finish line. They were okay, but were distraught about the bombing.

We continued our daily trips to Mass General until Friday, April 19, when the city of Boston, including our hometown of Watertown, went into complete lockdown while they searched for the two terrorists. We could not leave the house for our daily radiation treatments. I called Mass General to inform them of our dilemma. I thought the police would grant us permission to leave our home and go to the hospital, but that was not the case. Mass General told us to stay home because they were closing anyway.

Lynda and I spent the day watching the marathon bombing news coverage on TV, and for a while, we forgot about her cancer treatment and the impact of missing a day of treatment. At 6:00 p.m., the Governor of Massachusetts came on the air and told everyone that it was safe to leave the house. I took the opportunity to take the dog for a walk, and while walking on my street, I heard gunshots about two miles from my home. They found the Marathon Bomber. There was relief in the air, and then we went back to thinking about the disease and its impact on our lives.

Cancer impacts the patient, caregiver, and other family members, whether they live in the same household or not. As mentioned earlier, when my father was fighting cancer, I was a member of the immediate family but not living in the same home. My father's illness impacted me, but not to the same degree as it did my mother. Now, Maria was going through a similar experience with her mom.

Maria has provided moral and physical support whenever and wherever possible. She attended radiation and chemotherapy sessions and started a routine where she would text Lynda every night at bedtime and call every morning if she was not going with us to a doctor's visit. Maria could not do this without the support of her husband and children. This kind of support can be tremendous and infectious.

Friends and family can offer support, like grocery shopping, cooking dinner, or running errands for the family. Those were friendly gestures and helpful, but support also means more than that. Not everyone has the means to do these things; some people have physical or geographic limitations to help, but all of us can offer support and care regardless of obstacles.

A phone call to say hello can go a long way and sometimes means more than one's physical presence. When this kind of outreach doesn't occur, it can hurt and disappoint the patient and caregiver. Although at times we failed to understand this lack of outreach during Lynda's illness, we try to focus on the people in our lives who are positive, bring us joy, and reduce stress.

Consistent outreach by phone, email, or text can give a dramatic boost to the patient's mindset. The same is true for the caregiver. As the person who is there most of the time, you will see the patient's stress and endure most of the anger and frustration felt by the patient. Keep in mind that the anger and frustration you feel is not directed at you, but simply because you are there to receive it. It is a challenging position that you hold. You must grin and bear it. While it may seem like a burden, it is also a great blessing.

While you will sometimes feel the frustration of love *sought* and not *given*, you will also appreciate the love and support from those you least expect. These can be from friends, neighbors, work colleagues, or people with whom you lost touch but resurface at the right time. From these people, you can draw the strength needed to fight this disease.

When you offer help, the best example can come from giving your time and companionship—not something purchased. One of the most touching moments came on Christmas Day, 2016, when our eleven-year old grand-daughter, Abby, gave an exceptional gift to Lynda. It wasn't something that she saved for and bought, nor was it something that she made. It came from the heart with a message of love, support, and encouragement. Here's a small part of the note Abby shared with Lynda:

When my grandmother was diagnosed with thyroid cancer in 2013, we were all devastated. But each time she went into chemo, she was dancing. Sadly, she lost some of her hair and had a bad burn on her neck from radiation. Even so, she always maintained a positive attitude, which has impacted everyone around her. She keeps calm no matter what. Meemaw, we all love you so, so much, and no matter what happens, we will always be by your side.

My grandmother continues to put up a good fight and is doing an outstanding job. No matter what, she still goes to the beach and Cape Cod every weekend. Each day I spend with her, I treasure. She went through a couple of really bad times. I cried a lot during those times, but she was always there to comfort me and help me understand. She is my grandma, and I love her with all my heart. Cancer-free or not, Meemaw, you are truly my gift.

As a caregiver, I found that some don't like to ask how a patient is doing. They feel that they are intruding. The same is often true for the caregiver. My advice is to go with your instinct and do what you think is correct, but I suggest you err on the side of asking. If the caregiver doesn't want to talk about it, they will politely let you know by giving you short, one-word answers such as "I am fine" or "doing okay"—responses that do not typically encourage a follow-up conversation.

I have received many questions since Lynda has been in treatment; I can say that less than 10% are about the caregiver. And that is how it should be; after all, the patient is the person going through cancer treatment. But, the caregiver must seek and receive support because the caregiver must remain strong, clear-headed, and supportive.

So, when you have an opportunity to ask if a caregiver needs anything that you can provide, don't hesitate to ask. It doesn't have to be anything special or significant. It can be something simple. Meet for a cup of coffee and a conversation. Believe me, anything that can take the caregiver's mind away from the disease is helpful.

As you seek help, whether it's for you or the patient, don't be surprised if the person you contact does not show the same sense of urgency as you do. First, they are not as close to the problem as you are. They don't know what you face every day and may not understand your needs. Secondly, they may have a situation they are trying to deal with in their life. Even if they are close family members or friends, their needs will always come first. Understand this and try not to be upset by it.

The patient is under a tremendous amount of stress. The uncertainty of cancer can be devastating to a person's psyche. You need to find a balance between being supportive, doing all you can, backing off, and letting your loved one function as a normal human being. There will be a tendency to take over all the "chores" because you care and don't want to burden the patient with day-to-day stuff. Your efforts are admirable, but you may create a scenario where the patient will start to feel useless and unworthy. Knowing your loved one's normal behaviors and needs will help you identify the boundary of your support.

There will be times when you will get angry, frustrated, and, most definitely, lonely. It's okay and healthy to express these feelings by talking to someone or writing them down. There will be relief in expressing your emotions and realizing that what you feel is normal and completely justified.

As of the publishing of this book, Lynda continues to battle cancer, and I continue to do whatever it takes to see her through this. I am not alone, even though I often feel lonely. But I am strengthened by the belief that there's no greater purpose in life than answering the call to be a caregiver. No matter the outcome, caregiving changes your priorities and perspectives. The level of love, compassion, and empathy one feels while serving in this role has no limit.

Each day I get to sit by Lynda's side is a gift. I am grateful to the people who have helped me so far, but I am especially thankful to Lynda for entrusting me with her care. It is a partnership like no other.

I wish I could trade places with her—but I know that I can't.

 Husband to Lynda, father of Maria and Peter, and grandfather to Abby and Jack, Michael D. Tenaglia is a retired Bank Executive (CIO). A longtime member of the United Way of Tri-County, he twice served as Board Chair. Mike has been a community leader in the Greater Boston area for many years.

THIS PLACE ISN'T SO BAD

by Susan Scheer

Dad died unexpectedly in his sleep at seventy-seven years old. We were all devasted and stunned, especially my mom who had just lost her husband and best friend of fifty-four years. This was a profoundly sad and unsettling time for her and our family.

Once the shock wore off, our family's focus turned to taking care of Mom. I knew the day would come when our roles as mother and daughter reversed, and it was time for me to become her caregiver. My first concern was Mom living alone in a rambling three-story town house. She was starting to develop balance and mobility issues, so the thought of her going up and down stairs made me uncomfortable. Our family needed to develop a plan to ensure her safety and well-being. This was challenging because Mom did not see the need for a plan. She did not like or want change and was very comfortable in her current situation.

It was a blessing in disguise when some of her closest friends slowly started moving on and out of the neighborhood that she was living in at the time. Mom reluctantly agreed to start looking at new living arrangements. We started to explore all the various options that would be a good fit for her. This was a lengthy and somewhat excruciating two-year process because nothing seemed to satisfy her.

Mom finally agreed to move to a new housing development in the same town we lived in. She wanted to be close to me, my husband, and our daughter without living under the same roof. *But there was a catch.* She agreed to do this but only if we moved into the same neighborhood with her. After thinking this through, it started to make sense, so we decided to do it.

This was exhausting, time-consuming and at times frustrating, but we finally got Mom moved into her new "one-level" townhouse. We moved both houses in a few short months while my husband and I worked full-time and dealt with a teenage daughter who was having a rough time at school and struggling with anxiety and depression issues. It was the classic sandwich parenting dilemma, where you are taking care of your kid and a parent at the same time.

It took a while, but things calmed down. Mom eventually settled in and felt safe and comfortable in her new situation. She loved being close to her family. This made it all worthwhile for her.

For a few years, Mom lived a quiet, comfortable life. We realized we made the right decision for Mom and for us. It was so nice having her close—a two-minute walk from us. We could check on her often and turn on a dime if she needed help. Our family plan was working.

Mom's health was pretty good, considering she was in her early eighties. But then she developed a funny tickle in her throat that wouldn't go away. She didn't think too much of it but decided to go to the doctor to have it checked. Good thing she did because the little tickle turned out to be stage 4 lung cancer. All those years of smoking caught up with her, even though she quit in her late fifties.

This was a game-changer and one that impacted all of us. The doctor said without treatment, Mom had around six months to live. This was a terrifying moment, so we had to act fast. Mom agreed to radiation treatments but made it clear she would not do traditional chemotherapy. Then we learned about a clinical trial using a new immunotherapy drug, and Mom qualified. This treatment worked quite well and added an additional year and a half to her life, which was a gift to the family.

But eventually, the drug therapy was no longer effective, and Mom started to decline rapidly. She stopped eating and dropped weight dramatically, and her memory was fading fast. The doctor said there was nothing else she could do, so it was time to consider hospice care. Mom really wanted to die in her home. That was her wish—one that I desperately tried to fulfill.

The next few weeks were heartbreaking, tearful, sleepless, and extremely stressful. As her primary caregiver, I knew I was way over my head and needed professional help. Mom was going downhill fast, so I hired a hospice nurse and a few other caregivers who would check on her throughout the day and spend the evening watching over her. Mom's hospice nurse was a godsend who coached me, trained me, supported me, and even made me laugh. My priority was to take care of Mom and keep her comfortable while also juggling my own family and a full-time job. Looking back, I'm not sure how I did it. I have to give kudos to my husband, daughter, and brother, who all stepped up to help.

Mom was still living at home a week before she died. Her nurse was stunned at how rapidly mom had declined in just a few days. She clearly needed a higher level of care, and we agreed. It was time to put her into a hospice facility. This was the end of the road, and we knew Mom would not be with us much longer.

Twenty-four hours into her stay, she was in and out of a drug-induced coma but comfortable and in no pain. She was in highly competent and very caring hands. As difficult and sad as this was, I was relieved Mom was where she needed to be. In one of mom's more coherent moments, she looked at me and said, "This place isn't so bad after all." This was a huge relief and allowed me to step away from my caregiving role and back to being her daughter.

For the next few days, I sat bedside holding her hand and just chatted with her like old times. She was not able to talk back but could hear me and knew we were all there for her. She died peacefully, surrounded by her loving family.

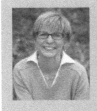

Sue Scheer and her husband John reside in Williston, VT with their rescue animals Lola and Ricky. They have one daughter, Kate, who is currently attending college in Fort Myers, Florida. Sue works full-time for Healthy Living Market.

THREE TO FIVE YEARS

by Linda Ronan

with Mark J. Resnick

My daughter was studying for her ordination exams when she first started to experience weakness in her left hand. She had trouble opening jars and then using a toothbrush, but she brushed it off because she lived a very busy life. A full-time mom, a soon-to-be-episcopal priest, a dog owner, and wife to a husband who was a full-time airline pilot. That was Jennifer Durant's life—and she loved it.

The symptoms were very gradual, and it didn't surprise me to learn she had ignored them for months. After all, her studies were demanding, and her stress level was usually pretty high. To her credit, she did give in to seeing an occupational therapist. The thinking was that maybe it was carpel tunnel syndrome and she just needed to strengthen her fingers and wrists.

In the meantime, she graduated from the seminary and was ordained a deacon in 2011. She received a job offer at the Church of our Savior in Charlottesville, VA, where she was to be the Associate Rector. Prior to starting the job, Jennifer and her family decided to do a bit of traveling, so they rented a motor home and travelled up and down the East Coast. It was a much-needed break from her hectic life.

Work started once the summer ended. Jennifer was still doing her carpel tunnel exercises, but they didn't seem to be helping with the weakness in her hands. That's when she decided to see a neurologist at the UVA Medical Center. I suspect she was doing some independent research on her symptoms and stumbled upon some articles that gave cause for concern.

She went alone to the appointment, and I pictured her wearing her collar, clearly a priest, with her blond hair and blue eyes. Jennifer was a beautiful woman. The doctor left the exam room and left her sitting there. She always had her bible, so she sat and read, worked on a sermon, and prayed. It turned out to be a long day. He was gone much longer than she expected. Two doctors came back into the room, and without asking anything about her or if she had any family along with her, they blurted out, "We think you have ALS."

"Ah, okay. So, what do we do about it?"

"Nothing. You have three to five years."

The UVA Medical Center chaplain on duty was actually one of Jennifer's classmates. In fact, he recommended Jennifer for her current job. The two of them took a long walk around the campus. Jennifer was distraught, but he encouraged her to remain positive, as much as one can after receiving a death sentence.

Her daughter, Kate, was eleven years old, and her son, Chris, was thirteen. Before calling the kids, she called my husband and me, and I believe her words were, "I *may* have ALS . . . but we aren't sure." We cried. We were destroyed.

Gradually, the symptoms worsened, but she was able to hide it from her boss for some time. It was much harder to hide it from her kids.

"Mommy, what's wrong with your hands?" Katie asked her.

In the winter of 2012, she told her boss about the diagnosis and volunteered to give up her position if she was unable to perform her duties. That wasn't necessary, he said, and so she stayed.

In the summer of 2012, Jennifer told the parish and her kids. I was a cat on a hot tin roof, waiting for her to share the news with Katie and Chris, but it was almost a non-event. Her family was a strong, Christian family, and the children had confided more in each other than we all knew. They may have been young, but they were smart and perceptive children.

After her fingers lost their strength, the disease took her hands, arms, legs, and finally, her voice. She went from using a cane to scooter to a wheelchair, then to something she called, "The Mercedes of wheelchairs!" I was going down every six to seven weeks for five-to-ten-day stays. Her husband, Matthew, quit flying; they gave him a leave of absence. He had caretakers stay overnight and get her ready for work the next morning. Fortunately, Jennifer was still able to work until ten days before she died.

Jennifer lost her voice in 2014. It was Easter Sunday. Her voice had been getting weaker and softer, then garbled and incomprehensible. Then, she could no longer mumble. The ALS Association was fabulous. The got her one of those Dynavox voice boxes, which gave her a "voice." It gave her so much joy to be able to speak with her family this way.

The parish and the school brought meals to the house. My visits became more frequent, as did the visitors, whether they were friends, family, or parishioners. She could no longer use the stairs, so there was always an extra bedroom for visitors.

Toward the end, in early February 2015, my sister Julie and I went down for a visit. We had planned to stay five or six days, but on the day we were supposed to go home to Boston, Matt asked me to stay longer. Hospice had been contacted, and they were handling her medications.

Jennifer had just delivered her final sermon a day or two before. She told her boss she was finished; she couldn't work anymore. She came home and sat in her chair with her favorite quilt and the cat sitting on her lap. Matt called us into the living room to tell us that mom was going to stop eating and taking her medicines. He told the kids she probably had ten days or a couple of weeks, then God would take her to heaven.

Matt pulled me aside and told me to go home for a few days. He wasn't kicking me out; basically, he was telling me to get myself together and come back at the end of the week. I wanted to stay, but my husband was home alone, and he also wanted to be with Jen.

Before I left, I sat next to Jennifer and held her head against my chest the whole day. In 2008, I had a mitral valve replaced in my heart. The doctors put in an artificial one made of titanium. It made this tick-tick soothing sound, and Jennifer seemed to like it.

My flight was early the next morning. I got home and gave the update to my husband. I went to bed early. I wouldn't see Jennifer alive again. She died on February 18, 2015—on Ash Wednesday.

Jennifer once told me that she was not in any physical pain—only emotional pain. She knew what was happening to her, but what was worse was knowing the outcome already. After the body fails, the breathing stops.

Her ALS course was pretty typical. They gave her three to five years to live, and that's what she got. She died on Ash Wednesday, and her parishioners made the comment that Jesus' ministry was within a similar timeframe before his death—three to five years.

"God didn't give me ALS, but he could take it away. Even still, I'd keep my ALS before I'd give up the blessings I experienced since my diagnosis."

I found it hard to accept her words, but that was Jennifer. She made extraordinary friends and had the most wonderful parishioners. The experience, in her mind, brought her ministry to completion.

Seven years later, I would be called again to be a caregiver. This time, for my husband, Skip. Like Jennifer, his disease—Parkinson's disease—was fatal.

Unlike ALS, Skip's Parkinson's symptoms were there from the beginning. I thought it was odd that he would forget my seventieth birthday, but there was a reason for that. He also became much more unresponsive during active conversations. Honestly, before we got the diagnosis, I thought he was just being a jerk.

I had told Skip for years to unload his HVAC company so we could have a life together again. It was all-consuming and causing all sorts of pain in his back. He had back surgery, but still, there was something else causing his absent-mindedness.

It was after the surgery in December 2020 that his doctors did the scans and saw that he had Parkinson's.

Caring for Skip is quite different from before. For starters, we won't be doing any more competitive ballroom dancing together. He's much more tied to the house than I am, but I can only leave him alone for around four hours. All of our doctors have told me to maintain my life and stay strong. Otherwise, I will be no help to him or anyone else. I've taken that advice seriously.

Caregiving changes how you see the world. We were devastated to learn about Jennifer's ALS diagnosis. Don't get me wrong—it was the most brutal experience of my life. But it also reminded me how precious each day is, how we need to be grateful for what we have—and mostly—to stop worrying about the small things that are outside of our control.

Linda has been retired since the pandemic and lives in Scituate, Massachusetts with her husband. They enjoy traveling, especially to see grandchildren and great-grandchildren. When at home, gardening is a favorite summer activity. Pilates and various forms of exercise take up the time year-round.

CARING FOR A CHILD WITH ADDICTION

by Art and Ginny Greenblott

with Mark J. Resnick

Our kids were born and raised in South Burlington, Vermont. It's the second-largest city in the state, but that's a relative number. When our kids were growing up, the city only had 10,000 people. It's doubled since that time, but it's still a wonderful place to raise children.

Wonderful but far from perfect.

Despite the smallness of Vermont—or perhaps even because of it—the state has some of the highest rates of substance abuse in the country, including higher drinking, cannabis and heroin rates for people aged eighteen to twenty-five. The only reason we're familiar with these statistics is because our family was part of them.

For most people, statistics are meaningless facts and figures. They're not irrelevant—they just lack personal connection or impact on most families. There's certainly no statistic in Vermont or elsewhere that shows one in four of your children will battle addiction. Even if there was, we wouldn't have believed it. But that was our reality with our youngest son, Brian, for more than twelve years.

Brian began smoking pot in the seventh grade. His grades started to go down for no apparent reason, at least none that we knew about. He obviously wasn't studying, but we didn't know why. The truth is, we were pretty naïve about the whole thing, but we had the "drug talk" with Brian. He was always such an easy-going, socially active kid. Everybody loved him, and he

223

got along well with his siblings. He seemed to understand our concerns, and we thought the issue was resolved.

But then in high school, Brian and a friend got caught smoking pot and were suspended. Thinking South Burlington High School may not have been the best fit or environment for Brian, we took him out and enrolled him at Vermont Academy for his final two years. It was a boarding school, but he seemed happy to come home on weekends. As we later discovered, he was only coming home to buy drugs so he could sell them at VA. Ultimately, he was caught smoking again; this time in his room, and he was expelled weeks before graduation.

VA let him graduate, thank goodness, but he didn't come home after graduation. Instead, he moved to Boston to live with his girlfriend, who was a schoolteacher. We thought she would be a good role model for him, and who knows, maybe she was, but during his stay with her, he started selling hard-core drugs. We figured this out when he showed up to visit us driving a BMW. My neighbor would comment, *There's something going on with Brian.*

Still, we dismissed it until one time Brian came home with a paper bag filled with a large amount of cash. He bought this massive safe and had it installed in our garage. That was certainly a red flag for us, and we became quite concerned about him. The worst was yet to come.

Between the ages of twenty to twenty-five, Brian was in the throes of selling and using hard-core drugs. There was one time when Brian tried to stop using drugs, but after a few days of not using, he became violently ill. He came home to see us and wanted to see the doctor. He also wanted to buy more drugs to stop the sickness, but we wouldn't let him buy any drugs. We held him down on the couch with the help of his sister, Kara.

We desperately tried to get Brian into rehab. Many times. We found a place in New York that would take him, and he agreed to go, which was a huge relief. But within a day of dropping him off, we learned that he left—he took a six-hour cab ride home to Vermont. He said he was scared; that all the patients were former prisoners from Riker's Island. His rehab stint lasted less than twelve hours.

Locally, we got him into Day One, an outpatient rehabilitation center. He lasted a few weeks, then quit. Over the Thanksgiving holiday that year, we held an intervention at his doctor's office. The whole family was present. Brian gave in, and we took him to a place called Maple Leaf. He did really well there and stayed clean and healthy. Until another relapse occurred.

Back to Maple Leaf, only this time he only lasted five days. Worse—he started hanging around with a bad crowd of people. We convinced him to try rehab again at the Betty Ford Clinic in California. An amazing place, but by the time we flew out to see him two weeks later for Parents Week, his advisor tracked us down to say that he was caught using drugs, and Betty Ford did not give second chances. They released him—the same time we were there visiting him.

Across the campus, we saw Brian walking away from us with a suitcase. We had no idea what would happen to him next. At the encouragement of the clinic, we stayed to finish our trip so that we could learn as much about addiction as possible. It felt strange to stay but so important to understand his world, our role in his world, and to cling to hope—to the possibility that our son could beat his addiction.

A few days after we returned home from Betty Ford, Brian showed up. Apparently, he had stolen one of our credit cards and flew home, but we did not allow him to stay. He moved in with a friend. One afternoon shortly thereafter, Brian was outside our front door. The rain was beating down on him, and we gave in—we let him come back—something you're not supposed to do.

We owned a flooring company and gave Brian a job. It seemed like a good idea. We could keep an eye on him away from his drug world. As it turned out, it was not a good idea. He often showed up to jobs high, though we weren't aware of this until much later.

One evening after work, I was driving up our street and saw Brian walking toward the car. He wouldn't look at me. When he did, I saw someone I barely recognized, as his face was beaten and bloodied. The people Brian used to sell drugs for said he stole from them—they were coming after him.

We called his counselor, who advised Brian should leave town. We sent him to Ginny's stepdad in Florida, who graciously accepted Brian into his home, knowing full well what was happening in his life. He threw Brian a lifeline.

Our son was no longer living in Vermont and had escaped the violence and danger of his drug community, but the addiction followed him. It wasn't until Brian was twenty-six that he began to take responsibility for his actions and attempted rehab again. I flew to Boca Raton to drop Brian off at Renaissance Recovery. He not only started a new program there but finished it. From Renaissance, he moved to a halfway house but still went to meetings. It was difficult, but Brian stayed clean.

Brian found work at a high-end office and retail furnisher company called Levinger's and became a department manager at their Boca Raton location near Renaissance. It was his first real job, and he worked hard. He stayed connected with Renaissance the entire time. For the first time in almost twelve years, we felt like Brian was on the right path. And he was.

We began seeing the old Brian again, and believe me, it felt like a miracle. Of course, we stayed on edge each time he called, always assuming the worst—another relapse. Fortunately, that call never came. When Brian asked us to invest in a new business opportunity—a tanning salon business—we did. It was a high-end salon, and although you could say we took a huge risk by putting some money into it, we didn't mind. It was worth it if it helped Brian stay focused and successful in this new life he created for himself.

Through his tanning solon, he got to know many of his clients very well. One in particular, another former addict, invited Brian to partner with him on a brand-new rehabilitation center. This time, the risk was all Brian's, as his potential partner told him upfront that he would not receive a salary until at least four months after the center opened. He said yes anyway.

Today, that same center is one of the largest and most successful rehab centers in Florida. In addition, Brian is a part-owner in thirteen halfway houses, another Wellness Center, and a construction company. He's been clean for twenty-one years, is married, and has a beautiful son.

It was a happy ending for us. We got lucky in that our son beat his addiction. But there's no hiding the fact that our lives turned upside down during those twelve years of active addiction. Not only for us but the entire family. All of our attention was on Brian. It was extremely difficult for our other children. Having a drug user in the house was not good for them, and it took a toll on everyone.

The choices we faced were terrible, and we made more bad choices than good ones. We enabled Brian. We bought things that he wanted, believing it would make him happy and remove his desire to get high. Our other kids resented the attention Brian received, especially Lisa, the sibling closest to him. We failed to acknowledge her accomplishments at every turn—not because we didn't care—but because we had focused so much time and energy on Brian and all the bad things he was doing. We didn't realize how badly we had ignored the needs of our other children.

His therapist told us, "He's going to get better, or he's going to die." That crushed our souls and clouded our judgement further. If a friend asked Ginny how she was doing, she would burst into tears. It wasn't until we attended the counseling program at Betty Ford that we received such honest feedback about parenting children with addiction: *Sometimes, the best thing to do is to do nothing.*

Easier said than done, right?

Ginny and I are very proud of Brian's recovery from addiction, but we're not so proud of how we handled his situation at the time. Lisa and Brian's relationship never stabilized, even today. That's on us. Both of us were naïve about Brian's addiction. He stole from us, came to work high, and pushed our family to the breaking point. Unfortunately, this is common within households dealing with addiction. To understand it, you have to go through it.

What most people don't understand is that drug addiction is just like any other disease. There are a variety of ways people become addicts, and it's easy to have a negative opinion of them. We used to categorize all drug users as weak, selfish, ignorant, or lazy. None of those things applied to Brian, yet, he became an addict. The disease is real, and there is no shame in talking about it. These people need help, not judgement. They need committed, caring therapists like Michael Herbert, who literally saved Brian's life when he first suggested we do a family intervention.

Caring for a child with addiction is an awful experience, but you can't come out of it without becoming a better person. It changes your perspective on life. It causes you to become more open-minded about people, their problems, and even some of the programs that can help them—or anyone—overcome massive obstacles, like addiction. For example, 12-step programs that teach addicts that in life, everyone tries to control everyone else, but the only person you can control is yourself.

The specific 12-step support program we became part of was called AL-ANON. Ginny has been attending meetings for the past twenty years, even though Brian has been clean and sober for twenty-six years. The support she received from that group made a big difference in her life and is the reason why she still attends meetings. When new parents show up with alcohol or drug addiction, Ginny can help them in the same way others helped her all those years ago.

Helping other parents deal with addiction is important to us—and it's hugely important to Brian. He knows where he came from and where he is now. As Director of Outreach for his rehab centers, Brian gets calls at all hours of the night. There's no sending them to voicemail or waiting for the morning. He drops everything, no matter the time or day, to help people fight addiction.

You can find information about AL-ANON and NAR-ANON in the Resources section of this book. If you have *any* concerns about a child, family member, or friend with a possible addiction, please don't wait to seek help or say something. It could quite literally mean the difference between life and death.

STILL WITH ME

by Laurie McLean

with Mark J. Resnick

My sister and I took my eighty-eight-year-old mother, Lucille West, on a cruise in 2005. The ship sailed to Key West, Honduras, and Cozumel. "Sprightly" is the kind word used to describe the elderly who can still function and enjoy life, and Mom fit that description. She required a wheelchair on the trip (just for safety) but did not use one at home, in her independent living apartment.

It was on the cruise that we noticed more subtle changes in our mom's health. Her voice was starting to get raspy. It was like she had a constant dry cough, but you could still understand her. We didn't pay too much attention to it—after all, she was eighty-eight.

Things changed the following year. The most noticeable feature about her that changed was her balance. Mom had very straight posture; she never hunched over and had remarkable strength for her age. She did her own grocery shopping and was very independent. Then the falls started, only she did a good job hiding them from us.

"Why do you have that scarf on?"

"It's nothing," she would say.

But we began to see the bruises on her neck and arms and started to worry about her overall health. Her reasoning was starting to diminish, too. She couldn't understand why doing certain things could be unsafe for her.

Something is definitely wrong.

The raspy voice on the cruise became raspier, so we took her to a voice specialist. We did everything we could think of to treat it, but nothing worked.

Yet the strangest behavior we noticed was how she often fell backward and for no apparent reason. She wasn't tripping; she was falling backward.

One particularly bad fall resulted in broken bones in her neck, which required months of treatment and therapy. Her health continued to decline. During one meal, she started to choke on her food and was rushed to the emergency room to clear her airways. This prompted Mom's move from an independent living arrangement to assisted living services. But even that wasn't enough care, as it wasn't safe for her to be alone any longer.

We hired around-the-clock care for Mom. Not only couldn't she be alone, but someone had to be with her while she walked, showered, and dressed to ensure she wouldn't fall backward and injure herself. The scariest development was her inability to sleep. Most nights, she literally stopped sleeping—maybe only sleeping thirty minutes a night. *This lasted for six weeks.*

Mom was showing signs of Parkinson's disease but without the shaking. We rubbed her legs and back and tried to get her into comfortable positions so she could get some rest. At work one day, I ran into a physician friend of mine who asked me about my mom. When I told her about Mom's lack of sleep, she immediately said, "You need to go see Dr. Singer. He is doing a sleep study and might be able to help your mom."

What a blessing that interaction was.

Two days later, we got her into the sleep study. Dr. Singer was so gentle and understanding. He performed multiple cognitive tests before diagnosing her with Progressive Supranuclear Palsy (PSP).

I had never heard of PSP, which is a rare neurological disorder that causes problems with movement, walking, balance, and eye movement. The nerve cells in the brain that control one's thinking and body movement are damaged. You don't lose your memory like Alzheimer's, but you do lose your reasoning. The disease is not well known, and it's unclear how those cells actually get damaged. We were told it could develop from a virus or be chemically induced, which made more sense, as Mom cleaned college dorms for twelve years and refinished furniture as a hobby for most of her life.

A neurologist confirmed the progressive supranuclear palsy diagnosis. There is no cure for PSP, and my mom was in her late eighties. When we asked the neurologist what we should do, he replied, "Just watch her every minute. Her food will need to be cut into tiny pieces to avoid further choking. Other than that, there's not much more we can do for her."

Mom had the most wonderful doctors. Knowing Mom couldn't be making frequent trips to the doctor's office, both her primary care doctor and the physician doing the sleep study came to her. They prescribed a low dose of Seroquel, an antipsychotic drug used for mood disorders, to help her sleep. Each week, they tweaked her doses until she was finally able to start sleeping again.

My family and I knew the next step would be a nursing home, but we promised to never do that. I know a lot of children make that promise to their parents or vice versa, but we had our reasons.

After one of her falls, in which she suffered a broken rib, she was sent to a nursing home to rehab the injury. The place was supposed to be the best one in Burlington, but Mom was badly mistreated there. The staff thought she was crazy because she had so much trouble speaking. My sister and I could understand what she was saying, but the staff couldn't—and never bothered to try. All she needed was help to the bathroom during the night. Instead, they put her in a wheelchair twice as big as the one she required, wheeled her into the dining room, and left her there for hours. She was put in a corner where she remained until 4:00 a.m. Although she couldn't speak, Mom was fully alert and had her wits about her. She tracked the time and told us about it—and we were outraged.

That's why we made the promise to never do that again.

When the disease progressed to the point where she needed more care or had to be placed in a nursing home, the staff at her assisted living home called a meeting with their entire staff. They knew her well and cared for her well-being, so they decided to allow Mom to stay at her apartment. She would need round-the-clock care and other arrangements such as a hospital bed, but they made it work.

I am the youngest of our six siblings and gave Mom the hard news: the disease was progressing, and nothing more could be done from a medical standpoint. But the good news, is that you can stay right here in your apartment—you are not going to a nursing home.

My sister Jackie and I took the brunt of shifts during the end of our mom's life. We were there most nights until 9:00 p.m. and spent much of our weekend caring for her. A week before Easter, I was feeding Mom. I say feeding, but it was only tiny spoonfuls of broth using a baby spoon. Still, the liquid gurgled in her throat as she was losing the ability to swallow. The next night, she went into a coma.

There are many universal experiences for caregivers when their loved one's life is near the end, and we had them, too. "It's okay to let go" was one of them, and we reassured our mom that it was, in fact, okay to let go. But she stayed in a coma for the entire week, until Good Friday. We arranged her room in bright Easter decorations, rubbed her arms, listened to her breathe, and swapped stories about her—we couldn't get enough of her. She was our rock.

At 8:00 p.m., the nurses came in to give her morphine and fluff her pillows. When they lifted her head, Mom's eyes opened. Tears came down her cheeks, and she looked at us intently. Her head couldn't move, but her eyes could. She couldn't speak but didn't need to. We knew she could hear us as we reassured her again, it was okay to let go and be in peace.

We talked to her until about 11:00 p.m. when her eyes got tired and were closing. Before leaving, we told her one final time: "It's okay to go, Mom." Jackie said, "It's time to fly with the butterflies now."

She died within the hour.

It was a beautiful death, and we were so grateful to have had those final hours with her. It was the ultimate gift by my mom, a person who had touched so many lives over the course of her ninety-one years on earth. She grew up on a farm in Canada and only had an eighth-grade education, but she impacted a lot of people.

The day after she died, the Nun who visited and took care of her asked us what time her eyes opened that night. After telling her, she said that's exactly when I was coming home from Good Friday mass. "Every light in my house was on—and I live alone. Lucille was trying to tell me something."

Emily was another of Mom's caregivers—one of her favorites. She was a family friend and college student getting her master's in psychology. These two were kindred spirits. Emily also asked about the timing of Mom's eyes opening. "I was in NYC getting on the subway at the time. There was a man playing *Amazing Grace,* and I started to cry because I thought of Lucille." Emily talked about Lucille in one of her psychology classes. Each week, they talked about Lucille. When the professor broke the news about her passing, every one of the students cried.

Lucille died in 2008, but she still comes to me. I learn things from her all the time. Something will come up during the course of cooking or gardening, and I'll say to myself, *Oh, that's why she did it that way.* Sometimes, I'll smell her, visualize her smile, or hear her laugh while taking a walk, and it immediately brightens my day. I think of her sense of humor, the honesty about her, and how humble and kind she was. Only she never knew it.

I'm a very independent and stubborn person—to a fault, quite honestly. When I was caring for her, I would not let myself cry. *OMG, how much longer can we go on?* I would say to myself. But I never let myself cry. I stifled it for two years, for I knew if I started, I wouldn't stop. The night she died, I finally gave in. I lost it. I cried so hard that hospice was comforting *me.*

Caring for Mom those final years was demanding, draining work, but I cherished every minute of it. I had no idea what a blessing it was at the time. I wish she hadn't gone through that hell, but we did our best to make the experience as light-hearted as we could. It was a privilege and honor to give my mom the care she needed.

Taking care of Mom also showed my two sons what it was like to care for someone you love. They were in high school and college at the time, but both were very good at helping out and spoke at her funeral. The night before her funeral, I was a typical mom, panicking that my oldest son would not be pre-pared for his talk.

"You need to write something down—have some notes."

"Don't worry," he assured me. "I will; I promise."

My son later told me what happened that night. He had started to write in his notebook but was interrupted by a knock on his door. He opened it, but nobody was there. At that moment, he knew it was Grandma—and he didn't write anything further down. According to him, "She had my back. I knew what to say."

And she did have his back. He delivered such an elegant remembrance.

About six years after she passed, I went to see a spiritual medium. *Yes, a psychic.* I wanted to connect with my mom, but mainly, I wanted to know if we did okay by her in the end. It was the biggest question on my mind. Taking care of her was indeed a blessing, but it was my blessing. I didn't outright tell the medium what was on my mind; that would be too easy, right? But in my head, I just kept asking my mom, *Did I do alright by you? Did Jackie and I take care of you?*

"Yes," the medium said after some long and awkward pauses. "Lucille is quite proud of you both."

I feel as close to her today as I ever have.

THE DIFFERENCE BETWEEN LIVING AND EXISTING

by Gayle Schreiber

I do not know where to begin. I am a caregiver, and yet I am not. In 2013, at eighty-five years old, my mother was diagnosed with dementia. My brother had moved back home with her in Philadelphia about nine years earlier after he lost his job. I lived and worked in upstate New York, about six hours away from my mother and brother.

After her diagnosis, I noticed that my mother was getting more forgetful, but they seemed to be doing okay. My mother still played word find games and solitaire and did some of the dishes. I did feel she was getting more isolated. I scheduled nurse's aides to come in twice a week to help my mother with her baths. My brother set out her medicine and prepared meals or ordered take-out like pizza, Philly Cheese Steaks, or Chinese food, working around my mother's kosher household. The Kosher Butcher also delivered prepared kosher meals like homemade soups or meatballs.

When I visited, I noticed a decline. My brother told me the aide was on vacation and would come while I was there. My mother stayed in her pajamas most of the time and did not get washed or dressed. When I took them out to dinner, it took effort to get her ready. She was very distracted, and I had to help her get her clothes on. I remember talking to my brother about it, saying that she might not even qualify for assisted living if she could not dress herself.

I knew my brother would not be able to continue to care for her if she got any worse or if his own health issues, uncontrolled diabetes, and heart and liver disease, declined. He assured me they were doing okay. There would be complications if we placed my mother in a nursing facility or memory care unit. In order to qualify for Medicaid, we would have to sell and spend down the cost of her condo, potentially leaving my brother homeless. Both their incomes were low; I needed to think about both of them.

I remember speaking with a few friends about this, saying, I need a plan B. What will I do if my brother passes away or becomes unable to care for her? It sounds cold, but in retrospect, I am pretty sure I should have done more. He was in over his head, and neither of them were in great shape.

Friends continued to assure me that it would probably be fine. He would say something if he could not care for her or if he needed help. Still, I started formulating a plan to move my mother up with me and look at assisted living and memory care facilities.

All hell broke loose on September 25, 2016, about four months after that last visit, when I got the phone call that my brother had passed away. The unthinkable had happened. I almost passed out and had to sit down. After a few deep breaths, I was able to compartmentalize and went into action mode. I didn't have time to grieve yet. I spoke on the phone with the policeman on the scene. They were getting ready to place my mother in a facility for the night, as I would not be able to get there until the following morning. There were no more flights out to Philly.

My mother's dementia had gone from mild to moderate instantly. She had seen my brother die, yet she could not remember it. She ran out and pulled the fire alarm, which alerted the fire department and police. I was able to get hold of a cousin who picked my mother up and took her home to his house for the night. He also helped me arrange a car rental and put me in touch with the same funeral home that took care of my father's arrangements.

First task: have a funeral service and bury my brother. Second task: start packing my mother up to move in with me and get a handle on her finances. Even though I had power of attorney, we hadn't discussed what she had for assets in many years. Third task: arrange adult day care or aides to stay with her when I went back to work. And many other tasks to follow, like taking care of my brother's estate (almost nonexistent but still a lot of paperwork), selling his car, selling my mother's condo . . . I was so overwhelmed.

Two weeks after my brother's death, my mother went looking for my brother in the middle of the night and fell. I do not know how long she lay there while I slept in the other room. I found her in my brother's room when I woke up early in the morning. I spent the whole day in the ER with her. They were going to send her home even though she could not walk. I finally got them to do X-rays on her pelvis and hips, and sure enough, she had fractured her pelvis in two places; we later found out she had a stress fracture on her spine. They admitted her to the hospital.

When I returned to her condo that night, I just sat on the floor and cried. I was grieving the loss of my brother, and I was grieving the loss of the mother who had raised me and was becoming a different person from the one I had known all my life. I was also grieving for me, overwhelmed with what had to be done and family-less except this stranger who was once my mother.

Despite my grief, having her admitted to the hospital was a blessing in disguise because she did not need surgery and was going into rehabilitation after five days in the hospital. I arranged a medical transport to a facility near my home in upstate New York. While she was in the hospital, I visited her for several hours every day, but I had time to sort out the packing, paperwork, and condo without the distraction of caregiving. I was able to sell her condo and the car. The closing was a week after she arrived in New York, which gave me time to complete packing and shipping her belongings and go through all her finances. I followed her back to New York a week after she left, right after the closing. I arrived home on her eighty-ninth birthday in late October 2016.

And here comes the second part of this story.

I had to decide what to do after the end of my mother's three months in rehab. My mother was borderline for qualifying for the nursing home but bringing her home was not an option because I was by myself with no family support. I was still working full-time. There was a bed in an assisted living facility, but she would run out of money after about a year. Her income was not high enough to pay the $6,000 per month for assisted living. She still had not shown me that she could dress herself.

Between my brother's death, the move to New York, and the fractured pelvis, my mother's dementia had gotten much worse. I made the decision to move her into the nursing home in the same facility as the rehab center. We now began our Medicaid spend-down—the point of no return.

It would not take long to go through my mother's life savings, and there would be no turning back once the spend-down was complete. The Medicaid paperwork was cumbersome with a five-year lookback. My mother was an accountant but had not kept any records or balanced the checkbook in the last five years. I had to go to all the banks, insurance companies, her pension, social security, etc., with copies of the power of attorney and get five years' worth of documents.

It surprised me that the federal government does not recognize the power of attorney, and of course, federal agencies do not talk to one another. I had to apply as a representative payee for her federal pension and social security, which required me to fill out paperwork annually for all the agencies to prove her income and how I spent her money. In the end, the application paperwork for Medicaid filled a four-inch, three-ring binder and took many hours of research and work to put together. All while I was working full-time.

During that time, as part of her spend-down, I paid for my mother's funeral and placed it in an irrevocable trust, with a copy in the Medicaid binder. It only took three to four months to spend down my mother's life savings. How sad is that?

I visited my mother every day until COVID-19 hit to make sure she was getting the proper care. On some visits, she would stay in her pajamas for the day. Sometimes her hair wasn't even combed. She constantly asked me where she was and when she could go home. She asked me to let dead people know where she was. Sometimes, I went along with her but felt like I was lying to my mother when I told her everyone says hello and made up stories. Sometimes, I tell her the truth that she has outlived everyone. It feels painful to me to watch her as she comprehends that everyone she knew and loved is gone.

Luckily, her short-term memory is so short that she will forget it in about twenty seconds. She has been there going on six years next week. I still visit her most days, although I now allow myself at least a day off a week. COVID-19 made me realize I was burning out.

My mother caught COVID-19 twice. *What a survivor.* She has also survived several falls since she got to the nursing home, once fracturing her arm, and once having a bleed in her brain. They called me at 3:00 a.m. to ask me to approve sending her to a hospital in the bordering state of Vermont, for brain surgery. Since she was almost ninety-five, I wanted to speak with the surgeons to see if people her age actually survived that kind of surgery. Their advice was to wait six hours and do another CT scan. I am glad we did because the bleeding stopped on its own. Because many of her aides tested positive for COVID-19, my mother was repeatedly placed in isolation, even when her COVID-19 tests were negative.

During one of my visits, after she was out of isolation, I got the virus and was sick for several weeks. I felt like I was putting my own life in danger just by visiting since they did not seem to control the virus very well in the facility. The isolation phase of COVID-19 brought her to the next level of dementia. I go to visit, and she no longer can find her words. She can barely walk and wants to sleep often. It breaks my heart over and over again. The worst thing of all I have been through is that I feel like I have placed my own mother in prison.

It haunts me every day.

Between the months of December 2022 and January 2023, I received twenty-two emails informing me of residents and/or staff testing positive for COVID-19. She loses ground every time she ends up in isolation. She can barely walk now and needs physical therapy because she sits in a chair all day. The pandemic might have entered the endemic stage for the general public, but it was still in the pandemic phase in the nursing home.

One thing I realized is that I am a strong person, and so is my mother. I had to accomplish and learn so much in a very short space of time after my brother's death. I get this from my mother. I just look at everything she has gone through.

It's been ten years since my mom was diagnosed with dementia. She remains in the nursing home. Earlier, I called my mom a survivor, and she is. But sometimes surviving isn't living—it's merely existing.

The woman I knew and loved and cherished my entire life is not recognizable any longer. I still visit her often despite her not recognizing me. I still answer her questions or sit in silence; I still hold her hand and kiss her goodbye.

She's my mom, and I'll always be there for her, but there needs to be a better ending for people with terminal diseases. The line between living and existing is a fine one, and I don't have the solution. But certainly, we can do better.

Can't we?

EVERY CAREGIVER NEEDS A CORNER MAN

by Brett Miller

The sounds of the ER at South Shore Hospital enveloped me—beeping monitors, hissing oxygen tanks, and busy but muted footsteps outside the private room. And the smell—that sterile smell we all know too well, no matter the hospital—never waned.

You were the best.

Those were the last words I said to my dad, as I held him in my arms, moments before he expended his final breath on earth. *Final permission given,* this proud Marine acknowledged. Not that he needed my permission, but I wanted him to know that it was okay to surrender to the overwhelming, complicated medical issues that slowly gnawed away at his body these last twenty years.

It wasn't meant to be this way, I kept saying to myself. Dad and I agreed we would utilize hospice services these final two weeks so that he could crossover in my home, surrounded by his loving family. We made this plan two weeks prior, following his ninth heart attack. I wanted him home with my wife and five-year-old daughter, Isabel. We wanted his final weeks of living laced with silver linings, resilience, grit, and pure love.

Dad's morning routine was methodical. To start, he consumed a large variety of pills, followed by his bowl of Cheerios, a banana, and coffee. He loved his first cup of coffee. He would then spend his day helping around the house, doing small chores, preparing meals with my wife, or watching countless Western movies starring the typical manly men: John Wayne and Clint

Eastwood. Sometimes, it was hard to believe that his time was coming—that his heart was failing him.

His favorite time during his final two weeks here on earth was the end of each day, around late afternoon. Typically, he would be posted in his recliner with the heating pad on his back and the foot pedestal up, catching the last rerun of *Bonanza*. My Isabel, just five years old at the time, would wrap herself up in a blanket and lay under or on his feet like a kitten or small dog nestling her master. Man's best friend. She would purr and meow as she snuggled him, keeping his poorly circulated, bluish, and leathered skin warm. He would talk to her like a baby kitten, and she would affectionately respond by cuddling. This mutual dance of true affection and bonding went on daily and for sometimes an hour.

Isabel still talks about these memories of her grandfather.

Yet when the all-too-soon-moment came, and my dad could no longer fight back against his shortness of breath and lack of cardiac output, our plan got nixed; instead, he took his final ambulance ride to the ER. I knew this was likely the last choice he would ever make on his own, and I honored it.

Those last two weeks were the most cherished hours, minutes, and seconds of time, not only for my relationship with my dad but for the whole family. The irony behind this special bond between us was that he was not my paternal father, but he was the only dad I ever knew, and he grew to be my best friend for life. He rescued my mom when I was seven and adopted my brother and me after they married. My mom had scraped together a life for us as a single mother, working two jobs day and night to make ends meet—until he came along and offered love, support, and a sense that everything would be okay for two young boys with no male role model.

Dad's time with us was one of the few instances I can recall that we truly lived in the moment. It was the greatest blessing, not only to have him in our home but also to be holding him during his final breaths in the hospital. So many speak of wanting that last moment with a loved one or just one more day, and I got the golden buzzer of a lifetime.

The highest honor one can achieve and have the opportunity to perform during life is the act and art of caregiving. To be so special that someone trusts and believes in you so much that they relinquish their health and safety to you when they are in their greatest need; to be in service to my dad throughout his last twenty years, but specifically, his last two weeks of life. What a blessing.

Life-changing, as you will see.

Despite the frequent storms that come with caregiving, and the array of feelings involved from fear, fatigue, frustration, and sadness, there are silver-lined blessings on the caregiver roller coaster. Some are realized in reflection, days after your commitment as a caregiver has come to an end. There is no textbook or research data for caregivers and every situation is like a snowflake falling from the sky, unique in its presentation and forever changing along the way.

Some days, you are tiptoeing through a minefield, and other days, you are celebrating small victories, like taking a walk in the woods by yourself or finishing a book that's been sitting on your nightstand for months. We do know one thing: caregiving takes endurance and can be very arduous and exhausting, physically and emotionally. But we also know that with the whirlwind of anticipatory grief and the mental warfare associated with being a caregiver, there has to be structured self-care time and support systems in place. In coming together during these times of adversity, our relationships with the ones we care for grow stronger with each passing day.

Your journey may start as a dedicated care partner to a loved one, where you and the recipient share a sense of purpose and play a specific role that is collaborative and cooperative. But it may also transition into a caregiver role in which your loved one is no longer able to care for themselves, meaning they can receive care but can no longer actively participate in their own care. Whether you are a partner or a full-time caregiver, both roles are essential in this journey.

How does one find wellness and support in the caregiving journey, so that they have a safe place to be heard, care for themselves, and find tranquility?

In 2017, I took a giant personal and professional leap when I founded and developed 110 Fitness, the largest wellness center in the world for people with Parkinson's disease. This was my silver lining and blessing from my caregiving days. Not only to offer a platform for people with chronic disease to break down barriers but also to offer a 360° platform for self-care and wellness for caregivers *and* care partners.

The mission of 110 Fitness was clear: leave no one behind and bring people back to life.

This had always been the mission of my eight-year commitment to the United States Army as a combat medic, and it would continue to spill over into my wellness center. Our programming initially consisted of boxing (non-contact), cycling, yoga, meditation, water fitness, and art workshops for Parkinson's patients. Yet it became obvious that there was this tremendous need to service our caregivers, too, many of whom had already begun to develop a pseudo-support group while their loved ones were in class.

My goal was to have the best facility in the nation available for our warriors, but also for their family members and caregivers, who, most of the time, were synonymous. This led to the creation of bi-monthly support groups and fitness classes for caregivers, as well as a volunteer program to educate them on the disease process, fall prevention, and the facilitation of movement techniques. Soon after, we developed a medical advisory board, which would include neuropsychiatry, community liaisons, and movement disorder specialists, just to name a few.

One unexpected blessing that came from our caregiving program was the opportunity to strengthen intergenerational relationships. Caregiving is a large team effort and requires the support of all family members, including children and grandchildren, who develop skills to cope, receive lessons on patience, resilience, and what it means to be in service of others. Beyond the family, Parkinson's care teams include attorneys, financial planners, social workers, chaplains, therapists, respite care workers, and close friends. We included them all in our circle of compassion here at 110 Fitness—it's what I like to call the Caregiving 110 style.

As our population of Parkinson's warriors and caregivers started to grow, so too did the strength and variety of our programming. Beyond the confines of our physical location in Rockland, Massachusetts, we now enjoy family time through bowling, golfing, musical concerts, rock climbing, axe throwing, movie screenings, orchestra outings, deep sea fishing, plays, art workshops, and more.

There are many amazing caregivers in our 110 Fitness world, but there's always a few that standout, who are deeply committed and go above the call of duty. These volunteers, sometimes called corner people at 110, are not only caring for their loved ones suffering from Parkinson's disease and its mental warfare at home, but also give their time in support of others at 110. They attend family support groups, exercise daily in our non-adaptive programming, and help with community event setup or drive our shuttle van to provide transportation for those in need.

One particular care partner who emanated courage and pure grit in the forever-changing Parkinson's journey was one of our spouses. From start to finish, as ugly as it became with her husband's mental status changes, multiple falls, and twenty-four-hour attention, she displayed pure love and true kindness in the very fibers of her soul. After the grueling end stages of Parkinson's and the loss of her husband, this woman—broken, dented, tattered—yet fiercely devoted to her husband, showed up in the much-needed walls of 110 Fitness to become a volunteer. There is nothing quite as remarkable as filtering through heavy sadness, grief, and the loss of your best friend by being of service to someone else in the struggles of a diseased life.

When I stop to digest the time commitment and emotional and physical endurance of these caregivers, I am profoundly touched, honored, and inspired. They command such gratitude and respect in the world of caregiving integrity. What a blessing it is to be surrounded by such human spirit on a daily basis.

Caregiving is the ultimate battle, but as long as the recipient of our care is willing to get in the arena and fight until there's no more fight to offer, it is worth it. My dad suffered through nine heart attacks in a twenty-year span, and I was blessed to be his cornerman during his battle. He truly was the best, yet, I am reminded of him each and every time I walk through the doors at 110 Fitness and see my Parkinson's fighters, caregivers, corner men and women, and extended family members. It is their perseverance, courage, resiliency, loyalty, strength, and honor that have made me a better coach, cornerman, and human being.

If you don't have a place like 110 Fitness in your life, find one. Caregiving isn't a battle that is best fought alone. There's no shame in asking for help. Check out the Resources pages in the back of the book, or call me personally. We will find you the help you need to get through this difficult time. You will not regret asking for assistance, and I say this from my own personal experience and from watching families struggle with Parkinson's disease and dementia every day.

Believe me when I say this: every caregiver needs a corner man or woman.

 Brett Miller is the founder and owner of 110 Fitness in Rockland, Massachusetts, the largest wellness center in the world for individuals with Parkinson's disease. A licensed physical therapist with 27 years of experience, he is a former U.S. Army veteran and author of the book, *It's a Beautiful Day to Save Lives: A Medic's Journey to His Destiny*, available on Amazon. Brett serves as the co-chair for the Massachusetts Parkinson's Registry as well as a Commissioner on the Massachusetts State Athletic Commission. He also serves as an ambassador for the Michael J. Fox Foundation for Parkinson's Research and the Davis Phinney Foundation. To connect with Brett, please visit www.110fitness.org.

DOING THE RIGHT THING

by Diana Peirce

"Cousin Stevie died late yesterday. He'll be laid out in the parlor for the wake, beginning on Tuesday," my grandmother said to me when I was seven years old.

This marked the culmination of the years of care my family provided to my then-six-year-old cousin—without comment or complaint (mostly)—like a fine orchestra performing a familiar concerto. Stevie's death also marked the beginning of celebrating his all too brief life, the courage and fortitude of his loving caregivers—all four generations—and the promise of "next time" because there would always be one.

As a child, I experienced caregiving firsthand in our traditional four generation household, all living under one roof. Direct care provision was usually the responsibility of the girls and women in the family, and extended family lived within a few miles of one another. Caregiving took many forms, including hands-on physical care, cooking (both for the ill person and those providing care), cleaning, laundry, financial and emotional support, and transportation—a seemingly endless list. Gramma called it "doing the right thing," and indeed it was.

My childhood prepared me well for assuming the role of caregiver and a lifelong career as a nurse in hospice and palliative care, as it turns out.

The role of caregiving is usually one of benevolent intentions and actions. Offering care to those in need is as old as humanity. Receiving care is often a humbling and, at times, difficult experience. The offering and receiving of care can be one of the most loving and grace-filled acts between humans. It can also be overwhelming, soul-deep fatiguing, frustrating, and all-consuming of one's time, energy, and finances.

Initially, caregiving may be born of adversity: an accident from which a loved one will recover in time, or a terminal diagnosis from which recovery is unlikely; or a child born with significant infirmities that will require a life-time of care and attention. All of these situations may result in an unanticipated caregiver experience, in which one is thrust into the role of caregiver. We humans have a marvelous capacity for flexibility and resilience, even in the face of unexpected and stressful situations.

But we are only human.

In his book, *Last Rights*, Vermont author Stephen Kiernan describes caregivers as representing "arguably the fastest growing component of health care," citing rapid hospital discharges (if patients are admitted at all). Caregivers are tasked with medical procedures such as changing dressings on surgical wounds, administering medications, and monitoring vital signs. He notes that this responsibility shift becomes even more pronounced at the end of one's life, when 24/7 care becomes necessary and the tasks of caregiving more numerous and complex.

This systemic change was initiated in the name of cost containment, of course, although many of us believe that care offered in familiar surroundings by familiar faces can result in overall better care. However, Stephen's point is well taken.

Caregiving for loved ones at home, whether recovery was anticipated or not, was once an expectation of family and friends. My own family of origin lived in a small section of our small town called the "Boro." Most of the homes of family members were located near one another. If out-of-town relatives or friends came to help, they were welcome to stay with another family member. Living in multigenerational households resulted in lots of teaching and learning over the years. Crucial tasks—assisting with personal care, bathing and dressing, preparing meals (especially for the ill person), administering medications, and still managing the household amidst all this—were handed down from generation to generation. We learned mostly by example, without a lot of planning or forethought. As Gramma would say, "It's just what we always did."

Contrast that with today's mobile society. Families are often spread across the country, if not around the world. Family members may feel ill-equipped to offer care, even if they're able to travel the distance to the bedside, taking time from their individual households and nuclear families, jobs, and other responsibilities. Some families are able to hire in home assistance, either privately or through an agency. The expense can be daunting, and the responsibility for overseeing such care is overwhelming.

Add to this the fact that siblings and other family members—often separated by time, distance, and temperament—are now expected to participate collaboratively in complex decision-making and to provide care about which many have little knowledge.

Daunting? Yes. Overwhelming? Sure. Impossible? Not at all.

In forty years of serving patients and their caregivers, alongside some of the most talented and committed professionals, I have seen fellow humans show themselves to be so resilient, rising to difficult occasions with grace and focus. Siblings who have not spoken meaningfully to each other in years present a united front of caregiving to an ailing parent. Those who can provide hands-on care. Those who don't feel they can provide financial and logistical support. Families divided by distance, circumstance, or misunderstanding come together for the first time in decades to meet a common need. And from that experience can come healing and hope.

As one son, the eldest of six, put it, "There's no rule that adult siblings even have to like each other, much less love and be present for each other, but at times like this, it sure helps. I think it was a comfort to our mom to see us working together after years apart. And in the process, we created new respect and healed some long-standing rifts between some of us. Will we all become best friends and find ourselves sitting in a circle singing Kumbaya? Of course not. But we were able to gain new perspectives and really see each other for perhaps the first time in years. I never thought I'd see Mom's death—and becoming an orphan at seventy-two—as a growth opportunity, but it was. And we seized the opportunity and made the most of it."

This family—they numbered at least two dozen individuals—was caught up for weeks in the day-to-day tasks of caregiving: personal care, meal preparation, and medication administration. Meanwhile, they were still able to discern and even embrace nuggets and moments of spirit-replenishing comfort, compassion, mutual gratitude, and understanding. In short, they were performing their own special concerto—a bit difficult, a little disjointed sometimes, a few "off" notes perhaps—but a piece unique to them.

Maybe that's the lesson in all this. We are wonderful, resilient beings, each with the capacity to share love, gratitude, and understanding, often in the most incongruent situations. Each of us has the capacity to share what we know, learn what we don't, and give from the depths of our being.

Each of us also has the responsibility to seek rest and sustenance when needed, as well as to sip from the collective cup of support and understanding. All this replenishes our capacity to offer care to those who need it. And as it was in my family of origin, there is always the promise of a next time, because there will always be one.

As Gramma wisely put it, "It's about doing the right thing." And I would respectfully add, "it can be so much more."

Diana Peirce has held hospice and palliative care leadership positions in Vermont, New England, and now California. Spanning several decades, she has published articles in several clinical journals, as well as editing a number of books, including clinical texts. Supported by her husband Tim, and their 3 children, her greatest joy has always been making a difference in another's life, sometimes through direct care, but often through teaching. A former lifelong resident of Vermont, Diana and her husband moved to Californian in 2010, where she continues her work in Hospice and Palliative Care.

THE INVISIBLE PATIENT

by Jamie Jacobs

As a clinical psychologist and director of the Center for Psychiatric On-cology and Behavioral Sciences at Mass General Cancer Center, I work with a team of professionals to provide accessible, state-of-the-art treatment for the psychological distress often experienced during and beyond cancer treatment. This distress extends not only to the person diagnosed and receiv-ing treatment, but to their family members who provide ongoing practical and emotional support daily, often at the exclusion of their own self-care. At the time this book is published, there will be approximately three mil-lion cancer caregivers in the United States. This number is rapidly growing as more people are diagnosed with and living with cancer.

Many people diagnosed with cancer will tell you that the mental and emotional aspects of cancer and cancer treatment bring about their own chal-lenges that are often left by the wayside. Difficulties with physical symptoms and changes in mood are felt by the caregivers as well, sometimes even more intensely. But we often aren't turning to the caregivers, the family members, to ask, *how are you doing?* It is no surprise that we aren't asking this question enough—we have few resources to offer family caregivers, due in part to a global shortage of mental health clinicians. To compound this public health problem, low reimbursement rates for behavioral health services force many clinicians to practice outside of insurance networks. As a result, affording a therapist and/or a psychiatrist is out of the question for those caregivers al-ready burdened by the financial toxicity of cancer and cancer treatment.

Caregivers are *integral* members of the oncology team, often tasked with providing care, ensuring medication adherence, and managing symptoms, as more medical care is delivered in the outpatient setting or at home (e.g., oral chemotherapy) and hospital stays become shorter. They are thrust into these roles with little information or preparedness and without much choice in the matter. Caregivers often selflessly give their time to caring, supporting, administering medications, and driving to and from medical appointments and procedures while managing their own jobs and other dependent family members and children. We hear directly from caregivers how they are stretched thin with little time to spare for themselves. It is no wonder we are learning that caregivers are experiencing more physical ailments, from colds to heart disease, as well as mood disorders like depression and anxiety. Caregivers are worn out and at risk for serious chronic illness and mortality, yet why are we not doing more for them? The physical and emotional burdens of caregiving have never been more prominent. In essence, the caregiver has become the invisible patient.

As Director of Caregiving Research in the Cancer Outcomes Research and Education (CORE) Program at Mass General Cancer Center, my mission is to apply our patient care model to the family caregivers so that caregivers can also receive support for the emotional sequelae that accompanies a cancer diagnosis and treatment. We are doing this by rigorously exploring the needs of cancer caregivers, adapting therapies that have worked to help patients manage symptoms of depression and anxiety, and testing these therapies in randomized controlled trials for caregivers. Learning practical skills to cope with distress can have a major influence on people's quality of life and their caregivers' quality of life. We are in the process of testing several therapeutic programs based in cognitive behavioral therapy, mindfulness-based cognitive therapy, acceptance commitment therapy, and relaxation training.

Some of these programs include one-on-one sessions with a caregiver and a therapist, while others are with the patient and caregiver together. Most of these programs offer between six to eight sessions, which are delivered virtually given the time constraints of caregivers and patients. The therapists focus on delivering practical, concrete skills for coping with stress, having meaningful conversations, managing physical and emotional symptoms with behavioral techniques, and helping caregivers find ways to prioritize self-care. We have already seen some of the promising effects of these programs on reducing anxiety and depressive symptoms and improving the quality of life in people caring for someone with cancer. In conducting this research, we are leading the way alongside several investigative groups worldwide that are committed to improving the lives of cancer caregivers.

We are working to help *you*, the caregiver. Our goal is to keep moving forward and build a strong evidence base for these brief, practical, evidence-based programs so that one day soon, they can be incorporated into the clinical care that we deliver. Personally, my goal is for every family member who walks through the door to be able to access supportive care services. To do this, I spend the better part of my days writing grants to fund more research or soliciting contributions to fund our research and clinical initiatives for caregivers. We do this because we need to make caregivers visible again.

We have had several caregivers who experienced the benefits of these programs, even noting that the skills they received have become like a guidebook for living their lives. The skills we teach our caregivers are very targeted and concrete. It's not like sitting on a couch and talking. We practice the exercises with them; we teach them how to relax and breath and be mindful of how they view stress. We give them the tools to cope and manage their stress, as well as a workbook that they can review. One woman told us that she brought the workbook with her everywhere she went. Here are some words from Michael Tenaglia, a co-author of *The Greatest Burden The Greatest Blessing* and a participant in one of our caregiving studies:

I'm so grateful I had the eight sessions with a therapist. It was an opportunity to talk to someone, to share my emotions—not just with a qualified person, clinically, but with a person outside the home. Sharing experiences with someone who is trained to help you. I know I wouldn't have received that support had I not been part of the program, so I would certainly recommend it.

The tools I learned allowed me to take a step back and take it all in. My therapist taught me not to take it so personally, whether it's the lack of support or a comment made by Lynda, my wife, for whom I am caring. If you can try and distance yourself from the situation at the right times, you might not get emotionally burnt out. It can get to you—cancer is difficult to watch happen. I've often turned back to the tools I learned to manage the stress. The breathing exercises have helped. Especially when you get bad news, and you're trying to process it all.

Caregivers all over should have the opportunity to receive this type of support that was so helpful to Michael. Our research program is one step along the way to making this a reality. The needs are enormous. There are more and more people living with cancer and, therefore, more caregivers. People are receiving cancer treatment for longer, so caregiving responsibilities persist and grow. We must find ways to make supportive care available to cancer caregivers and easily accessible. Caregivers deserve their own support systems and to prioritize their own self-care, both for their own benefit and the benefit of the person with cancer. If you are a caregiver, ask questions about where you might be able to get the support that you need. Caregiving might be a burden for you, or you might derive great meaning from this role.

Either way, you are not alone and might benefit from talking with someone to help improve your quality of life and manage stress. You are not invisible.

If you want to learn more about our Caregiving Research Program at Mass General Cancer Center or support the growth of our research and clinical programs, contact me personally or visit our website: *https://because.massgeneral.org/caregivingresearch.*

***

Dr. Jacobs is an assistant professor in the Department of Psychiatry at Harvard Medical School, a clinical psychologist at the Massachusetts General Brigham Hospital (MGH) Cancer Center, and the program director for the Center for Psychiatric Oncology & Behavioral Sciences. She is a clinical researcher, the director of caregiving research in the MGH Cancer Outcomes Research & Education program, and the director of research for the American Psychosocial Oncology Society. To donate to her research, visit because.massgeneral.org/caregivingresearch.

ALL FIRES BURN OUT

by David Traub

It will end.

There will be a last night that you stay up until 4:00 a.m. when your spouse rises to hold the baby, who cannot be left alone. A last night you sob from sheer exhaustion.

There was a last meal I cooked for my mother. Then a last time I helped her sit up in bed. There was a last frustration I resolved for my father.

For most caregivers, there will be a time after.

There was a last time I wheeled my grandfather around the nursing home. There was a last time I brought my guitar to play him songs written before I was born. A last time I sat by my grandmother's bedside to sing softly. Or pray in French, her first language, as if she could hear that any better.

The caretaking I have done is far short of what some have given, and more than others. You may find the same is true for you. But the dimensions, even the duration, of the gift you have given to someone that you have cared for is less relevant than the space it occupied in your life.

There will be a night you fall asleep without having to set an alarm to administer pre-dawn medication. A morning when the normal hour comes and goes with you still in bed, turning over rather than rising to serve. Or maybe you will finish a whole meal while it is warm. The relief may come in a whisper or a rush.

Some part of you may feel guilt at the relief, if that relief comes because your person's situation got worse rather than better, or maybe even ended. An emergency physician once told me: "All bleeding eventually stops." Some sense of guilt may be unavoidable, but I found it important to recognize it for what it was. We spend weeks or years of our lives caregiving because we

255

understand that love is an action, or sometimes it is a body of little actions strung together.

It is never free. Not to us. I tried to absorb the cost without counting or thought of reward. The return I got from that sacrifice of time and gift of love was intangible and hard to articulate. We will miss the giving, being the giver, even as we walk without the familiar weight on our backs.

Mémère is the *Québécois* word for grandma, and I was holding my *Mémère's* hand on that day, 102 years and two months exactly from when she first saw light. I was the first one who spoke after her last breath. The one who stayed with her until the men from the funeral home arrived because I did not want her to be alone.

As I sat beside her, I thought about her daughter, my mother, who was twelve states away when the urgent call came. And I thought about her late husband, my grandfather, who spoke his last word aloud to me in the emergency room following the stroke that would cost him control of his legs, his writing hand, his speech, and much more.

I had followed his ambulance to the hospital with my grandmother beside me in the front seat that day. When it was clear, hours later, that he was staying at the hospital and we had to get my grandmother home, it was me who walked in to explain to my grandfather what was happening. I told him he had experienced a stroke, and they would not know how bad it was for a while. But he was safe where he was, he would be staying, and however long it took for him to get better, I promised him, "We will take care of *Mémère*."

He nodded his head and said his last word, "Okay."

He would live another three torturous years, fed by a tube and suffering pain and silence as well as suffering my guitar playing. My *Mémère* would see another sixteen—most of them vibrant and independent.

During those sixteen years, I would change jobs, careers, cars, and addresses. I would advance from my twenties to my forties and get married to someone I trust and deeply love. I called her as I drove away from the nursing home that I would never visit again. I had been stoic without having to force myself to be stoic. Then the love of my life said, "David, you kept your promise to your grandfather." I was stoic no more. I felt victory and loss tossed together like vinegar and oil. Pain and honor and pity and love and sacrifice. Some of those emotions leaked out of my eyes.

When the end of your caretaking comes, you may find that you have kept your promise to yourself, or your spouse, your parent or grandparent—the one you love. There is no right way or wrong way to feel it. Don't chase it away. And don't be shamed by the pain or the relief.

Just know you kept your promise, above all, to yourself.

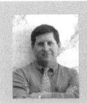
David's writing has appeared in dozens of publications, including freelance work at the Providence Journal and as a staff reporter and columnist at the *MetroWest Daily News*. Since reporting, David has worked in government, non-profit, and political communications. David continues to edit his first novel. Reach him david@davidtraub.com.

ON CAREGIVING

by Matt Perrin

"**M**att, your mom has Alzheimer's."

Those words changed my life. They made me a family caregiver, gave me a new personal and professional purpose, and unlocked a passion for helping others who find themselves in the position of caring for a loved one.

My mom, Rosemary, passed away from Alzheimer's in April 2022 after living with the disease for eight years. She lived a good life. Mom worked tirelessly as a widowed single mother to raise me and somehow managed to be the life of the party along the way. While Alzheimer's disease was a cruel and uninvited guest in her retirement years, Mom set an example of how to laugh, love, and live in spite of it.

She did that until she couldn't anymore and eventually became collateral damage of our country's broken long-term care system. Within four years, every penny of Mom's life savings was gone, all spent on the care and supportive living arrangement she needed because of Alzheimer's. When her money was gone, she was too—forced to move into a less supportive environment because she could no longer afford to pay.

Mom left Cape Cod, her home of thirty-two years, for the last time on September 9, 2021, while still ambulatory, verbal, and full of life. She would spend time in six different facilities over the course of the next six months, due in large part to a pervasive lack of dementia training throughout long-term care and a system structured to transactionally treat conditions instead of truly caring for the people living with them.

I'm eternally grateful for the kindness and compassion shown to her by many staff members at various facilities and recognize that they have impossible jobs because they're set up by the system to fail. Or they're not invested in such that they can succeed. Either way, the result is the same.

As my mom drew her last breath, she was three steps away from a leaking sink and broken dressers, and a literal arm's length away from her concerned and confused roommates—Ruth on the left and Arlene on the right—separated only by a curtain that hadn't seen a washing machine in at least a decade.

If Mom was still here and cogent, she would think nothing of her own circumstance and say something like, "I was one of the lucky ones." She would also be appalled by the quality of life provided to her fellow residents in their respective final days and how badly the long-term care system is failing our most marginalized and vulnerable. And she'd let the world know it.

Because that's who my mother, Rosemary Perrin, was.

As her only child and primary caregiver, those years were the darkest of my life. The extraordinary sense of responsibility, guilt, fear, exhaustion, anger, and sadness often consumed my entire being. When I emerged on the other side of that period of my life, I was a completely different person.

In the midst of the darkness, there was light. Over the course of her illness, the depth of our relationship went to a place that I never knew was possible. We were always close, but the more she sunk into her own world, the more reliant she became on me and the closer we became. There was a bond between us that was something more than sacred, even during the silence. And over time, I learned to see, appreciate, and cherish the beauty in that.

Mom raised me right. But it was the experience of caring for her that allowed me to truly bear witness to kindness, empathy, and love in their purest forms.

Her illness and our shared experience living through it showed me the importance of being present, of being able to see what's most important, and of paying those things the attention they deserve. Mom's illness showed me this in a way that words never could.

There's something else that happened along the way. Walking with Mom through her journey with Alzheimer's left me with a new brand of confidence. It's not a bravado laden, strut-my-stuff kind of confidence. Nor is it sheer will or brute force to "do anything I set my mind to." It's a subtle and quiet comfort that I take from knowing just how resourceful caregiving made me. And it benefits me in every aspect of my life.

When Mom's journey with Alzheimer's disease was beginning, my father-in-law, Steve, was beginning his own journey with Lewy Body Dementia. My wife, Lindsay, and I were fortunate—or unfortunate, depending on one's perspective—to walk this road together and simultaneously. While I spent years in the camp of seeing the timing as unfortunate, I came to see the benefit. We had the built-in support of each other when many don't. Better yet, we learned more than we would have otherwise because we had two experiences to learn from. And we share a determination for paying that forward.

To that end, in September of 2021, we created a weekly newsletter for family caregivers. We're experts in nothing but our own lived experience caring for our parents, yet we deem that experience worth sharing. Every Thursday I send an email with three things I've been thinking about, using, doing, loving, or hating in the caregiving week gone by. Because hearing and learning from other family caregivers was *the thing* that kept us going.

I was asked to share some posts for this book and hope you find them helpful.

***

Friends and caregiving

I remember being hurt and angry back in the early days of our caregiving journey, by friends who had seemed to disappear. They vanished.

I couldn't believe it, and I was hurt. Looking back on it now, though, I don't harbor any ill will or really even blame them.

If I did, that'd be like me saying that I would've kept calling a friend or inviting them to things after they'd declined or been unresponsive time after time after time.

I like to think I would. But I can't be sure.

So I don't blame them, and I'm not mad. Anymore.

Back then though, the loss definitely stung for a bit. It fueled my fear of missing out and gave birth to my earliest bouts of caregiving resentment.

But it was short-lived in the grand scheme of things—because of those who kept showing up and the new friends who came into our lives.

They were godsends.

Looking back now from the other side of it all, I can't imagine it any other way.

And firmly believe that it all worked out in the end.

***

People want to be good

I noticed a new behavior somewhere in the early to mid-stages of Mom's experience with Alzheimer's disease.

She'd begun reading things aloud. A lot.

Mom was always a reader. But not like this.

In the car, she'd read every road sign.

Walking into an appointment, she'd read every sign on the wall.

Waiting for that appointment, she'd read the cover of every magazine.

I can still hear her loud but uncertain voice.

I can still feel her pause after each sentence as she geared up for the next.

I can still see the look on her face that asked *am I doing it right?* And I can still feel the warm glow of her sheepish smile when she realized she was.

It was so interesting.

Kind of sad, too.

But most of all, it was good because it made her happy. Which brings me to the thing I wanted to tell you about.

Mom was in the morass of the long-term care system at the time. And I was jaded (understatement) by, well, everything and everyone. It was a dark time.

But then I saw this tweet from a marketing executive who I follow on Twitter named Amanda Natividad.

Amanda Natividad @amandanat · 1h

One of the mentally healthiest things I've done is to assume positive intent — that people are good, they're trying their best, and they mean well.

I am rarely proven wrong.

It got me thinking.

Assume positive intent.

People are good.

They're trying their best.

They mean well.

Assume positive intent.

The more I thought about it, the more I realized that I was so exhausted from assuming and thinking the worst about everything and everyone all the time, that I had to try it out for myself.

So I did. I tried it.

Better yet, I stuck with it.

Yeah, I'm proven wrong sometimes. But in general?

I feel lighter.

And I feel happier.

If you already do this, disregard it (and I'm jealous because I wish I started a long time ago).

If you don't, give it a shot.

It's worth it!

***

Worth remembering

It's another thing that I needed constant reinforcement on. I had to remind myself of it after Mom moved into a memory care community. A lot.

Maybe you do, too. So here you go.

Living under a different roof than the person you care for doesn't make you any less of a caregiver.

***

How can I help?

It used to drive me bonkers when people would say, "Let me know what I can do to help."

I knew it was meant well. I mean, sometimes I think it was hollow, but for the most part, it was usually always meant well.

The problem was that in those moments, I didn't know what I needed help with. Even if in my head I was thinking, *Gosh, wouldn't that be nice.*

I was so in the caregiving weeds that it felt like work to find something this well-meaning person could help with. Shoot, it was work.

So that's where this very sophisticated tip comes in. And like anything I share here, it came originally from someone else who offered this suggestion to me. It's another one of the countless tips and tricks I was lucky to learn from other caregivers I met along the way.

Anyway, the tip is *to make a specific list of needs.*

In calm caregiving times, sit down and write down a few specific things you need help with.

I need help getting Mom to the doctor on November 7 at 10:00 a.m. in Hyannis.

or

Tuesdays are especially hectic, and I never have time to even pick up takeout, never mind cook. I need dinner on Tuesday, and a burger would be fantastic.

or

Getting Mom out of bed is too hard for me to do alone. And it takes too long. I need help with that.

It can be one thing to start. Or a few things. Or a bunch of things. It doesn't matter.

What matters is that you start the list. And keep it handy. I kept it folded a bazillion times in the corner of my wallet.

So that when someone would ask, I would have specific things I could use help with at the ready.

And I'll never forget the first time I whipped it out. My mom's brother gave me the dreaded "If there's ever anything you need, just let me know."

The surprised look on his face when I said, "Actually, hold on a sec" and pulled out my list was pretty priceless. But even more priceless?

Him doing the thing that I needed help with.

***

Traveling with Mom

I'm not talking about "get on a plane" or "long car ride" travel here. That kind of travel was an entirely different kettle of fish kind of hard—which, at a certain point, became not worth it or not possible or both.

I'm talking about short travel around town. To appointments or activities—daily life. And because of Mom's Alzheimer's, even that became increasingly difficult.

The actual logistics (getting in/out of the house, getting in/out of the car) became more and more labor-intensive over time. I expected that.

What I didn't expect was how hard it was to have Mom simply sit in the car and be along for, or even enjoy, the ride.

She was cold. She was hot.

She didn't know what to do with her hands.

She was unsettled, which often led to agitation.

I didn't see this challenge coming, and it frustrated me to no end. But once I was able to step back, see the situation for what it truly was, accept the reality, and adjust my expectations accordingly—we got through it.

And two simple things really helped.

First was Mom's music. It was usually an instant soother.

I started with Mom's favorite radio stations in my car's pre-sets but then noticed whenever commercials were on or the DJ was talking instead of playing music, Mom would be antsy.

So, I made a Spotify playlist that I'd be sure to have ready whenever Mom was in the car.

Mom's music quickly became a must-have on any car ride—no matter the distance.

The second simple but helpful tool was a go-bag that I kept in the car. For me, it was just a big reusable shopping bag full of stuff that Mom liked or stuff that we might have needed.

A blanket

A small pillow

A fidget blanket

Assortment of snacks

A big bottle of water and a travel cup

A few old *People* magazines

Extra socks, undergarments, and bathroom supplies

Like everything else in caregiving, I wouldn't say traveling around town was easy. But the combo of Mom's music and the go-bag sure made it a lot easier.

I think she even enjoyed it at times.

***

Expectations ahead of time

This could come in really handy at the holidays or anytime family/friends will see your loved one for the first time in a while.

Give the friends/family a heads-up on what to expect beforehand. For me, it usually went something like this.

Hey so and so,

Mom and I are looking forward to seeing you on Saturday. Just wanted to give you a quick heads-up on a few things ahead of time.

You'll probably notice that Mom's speech is different—slower and softer—and she repeats the same statements and questions pretty consistently. A lot more so since the last time you saw her. Also, Mom gets really quiet at times, but that doesn't necessarily mean she's not enjoying herself. Her appearance has changed too (her hair is longer, and her skin is pretty pale).

This is all part of her disease progression, but I wanted to let you know in advance so the focus can be on including Mom in conversation, etc. vs the surprise at how she looks or is acting. If you have any questions, please let me know.

And like I said, we're excited for Saturday. See you then!

Sometimes I might even include a recent picture.

Doing this helped in a few different ways. It gave the family/friends a preview of what to expect and some time to process in advance.

I also found that it prevented some (some, not all) of the questions/comments that do more harm than good to me and Mom, regardless of the helpful or curious intentions. If you're a current or former caregiver reading this, you know the ones.

Finally, it proactively alleviated some (some, not all) of my anxiety about the visit.

So, if you're like me and get stressed and anxious about seeing other people with your loved one, this is worth giving a shot.

***

A "hack" that helped

Scanning documents with my iPhone is a small thing that I was late to the game on, but wow, has this been a game-changer for me. No more fiddling with our dated all-in-one printer/scanner or driving to Staples to make copies and scan.

Now all I have to do is:

1.   Open the iOS Notes app > Tap on the new note icon in the bottom right
2.   Tap on the camera icon > Scan Documents
3.   Put the document in question in the frame > hit the circle button > Save

The best part is that all of the scans stay in the Notes app unless I delete them, effectively turning my phone into a mobile caregiving binder, with signed versions of important documents like a Healthcare Proxy or Power of Attorney (POA) always at my disposal.

This makes the administrative aspect of my caregiving life so much easier.

***

You can subscribe to *Three Thing Thursday *on caregiving* by visiting www. threethingthursday.com/newsletter. It's free, and I don't profit from the site; it's simply a way for us to pay forward the comfort, validation, support, and guidance we've gotten from others along the way.

MOVING ON FROM CAREGIVING

by Nicole Danielle Bell

"Hey, Holly, what's up?" Holly was the executive director at Brookhaven, the resident care facility that housed my husband, Russ. She was always pleasant and helpful, but getting a call from her still felt like being summoned to the principal's office.

"All is okay. I was just wondering if you're coming here today. I'd like to chat about something."

"I'm on my way now and will be there in about five minutes. Do you want me to stop by your office when I get there?" I asked.

"That would be great. I'll see you in a bit."

I hung up the phone and made the last few turns into the facility, a routine I repeated four to five times a week. My first tour was still fresh in my mind—the smells, the vacant stares, the remnants of life. I'd gone home and cried for over an hour. But being there all the time, I saw the life and happiness that coexisted with the despair. Residents became friends, and I learned their stories from conversations with them or their family members. Each of the fifty residents had their lives, their family, their loss. The cost of Alzheimer's became more apparent with each new encounter.

Holly's office was the last door on the right before entering one of the resident wings. I knocked, and she invited me in.

"I have to admit that I'm nervous," I said. "You're great and all, but your job typically isn't sharing the good news."

She laughed. "Everything is fine. Russ is doing great. But I did want to tell you that he's been spending a lot of time with Daisy lately."

Daisy was a new resident in Russ's hall. I'd spent several hours with her on the outing to the State Fair and found her very sweet. Despite that, I knew what Holly was insinuating. It was the dirty little secret of memory care, or probably any assisted living. Men were in short supply, and when a new one showed up, there was no shortage of suitors. Of course, they didn't tell me that when I considered placement. I learned it the old-fashioned way.

It didn't take long to figure out the dynamics of the dementia dating scene. My indoctrination occurred during my second visit when I met Priscila. We struck up a conversation in the little coffee shop at the edge of the main meeting space. She introduced herself as Arthur's wife. Wait, what? Arthur's wife? Isn't Arthur married to Sally? I was smart enough not to say it aloud, but it took me a while to process the confusion. Then, as Russ and I drank our coffees, I watched the strange thruple share a snack at a table a few feet away. Sally was the Brookhaven wife; Priscila was the actual wife. I sat mesmerized as I watched Priscila handle the situation with remarkable class and dignity.

I wasn't sure if Russ would be interested in such a relationship since the early onset of his dementia meant that most of the female residents were much older. Initially, he struggled with me not being there all the time. When I left, he got angry and caused a scene, and one of the managers had to intercede to calm him down. But after almost four months, he was accustomed to his new home. I often found him in the living room with Daisy as they laughed and told jokes. They were inseparable, moving from space to space, enjoying each other's company. I guess the relationship wasn't as platonic as I thought. My suspicions were confirmed by Holly's body language.

"I see. What's been going on?" I asked.

"Well, at night, he often ends up in her room. It seems to be becoming a thing. I don't think anything sexual is going on, but we wanted to let you know in case that changes."

"Wow. What's your policy on that?"

"When we see something, we separate them and notify the families, but that's about it as long as it's consensual."

I attempted to navigate the uncharted territory. "And what about Daisy's family? Are they okay with it?"

"Yes. Daisy likes companionship, so they weren't surprised that she sought someone here. They're fine."

I took a minute to process. "Well, if you all are okay with it, and Daisy's family is okay with it, then I'm okay with it. Seriously, I just want him to be happy."

"That's a great way to look at it. If anything changes, I'll let you know."

On my way out of her office, I turned and laughed. "I don't think I realized the intricacies of your job until now. Damn, girl—life must get interesting."

She laughed. "You have no idea."

That night, after I put our two young children to bed, I relaxed into my new reading nook, a little alcove on the side of my bedroom with a cozy chair and a rarely used fireplace. It used to have two chairs, but one of them went with Russ to Brookhaven, so I rearranged the furniture and decor to claim the space as my own. Instead of picking up my book, I sat back and thought.

Okay, Nicole. What do you honestly think about this? It was weird, but everything about my situation was weird. It was a dementia unit. Daisy wasn't a home hussie. She was a sweet, wonderful person who was someone's mom.

A sharp resident at Brookhaven who was there only to help care for her husband filled me in on the whole situation. "You know, she sits with us at meals. She talked about Russ, and I reminded her that he was married. She looked right at me and said that she knew that because he was married to her." She chuckled and went on, "Then I told her to stay the heck away from my husband."

Daisy probably did believe Russ was her husband, and despite all my time with Russ, I had no idea what he thought. Some days he seemed okay, and other days, he had no idea where he was. I couldn't begrudge either of them for the situation.

Dig deep, Nicole. What do you feel? I dug, and I realized all I felt was relief. I prayed that Russ would find peace and dignity in the rest of his journey. What was better peace than the comfort of companionship? The man I

271

married had left us long ago, and the man that now existed needed a presence I couldn't give. Daisy wasn't a threat; she was an enormous gift to both of us. The guilt barraging my conscience eased, and for the first time in a while, I felt free.

With Russ moving on in his life, I realized I also needed to move on in mine. The kids consumed a good chunk of my days, but the evening hours became mine. When Russ was home, if I went anywhere or did anything, he followed. So, for him to sit, I had to sit. The logical answer was to watch television. Now, as I watched TV by myself, I discovered that I hated TV. Countless hours staring at a box with nothing learned; it wasn't how I wanted to spend my time. I had a free license to do whatever I chose, whatever I wanted. I soon discovered I wanted to organize.

Months and months of Russ's disease reaped chaos throughout the house. He emptied the contents of file folders for sport. He hid trinkets in mysterious places to keep them safe. He disassembled tools and separated their parts to obscure the source. Night after night, I picked a project and brought order to the pandemonium. I mentally inventoried and found logical homes for each item, often heralded by the help of my new coveted label maker.

As the clutter cleared, I moved to more significant projects I'd always wanted to tackle. My closet housed outfits I'd purchased decades ago and was ripe for a good cleaning. I culled and consolidated, but it still seemed cramped and messy. Then I walked out of my closet and stared at the two Scandinavian-style dressers in my bedroom. Since my closet was larger, Russ used both dressers for his clothes. They were his, even before we got married.

I couldn't use them, could I?

I walked by and straightened some towels in the bathroom, clearly delaying the looming decision. Soon, I was back, staring, almost paralyzed.

They're only dressers. Why am I making such a big deal of this?

They were only dressers, but they were his dressers. Some part of me still felt like he would come home and wonder where I put all his stuff, maybe even be angry. But the logical part of me knew that would never happen.

One by one, I emptied each dresser drawer and examined the contents. I found rarely worn clothes, old sweatshirts, out-of-style biking shorts, and scratchy T-shirts that never got worn. But there were a few finds that reminded me of who he was. There was the ridiculous Mao Tse-Tung watch that he bought on his first trip to China. It had a regal image of the leader with his hand pulsing over the crowd, each wave announcing the passage of a new second. Russ laughed every time he ran across it and occasionally wore it to see how people reacted.

Then there was his old tape recorder. Back when we first met, before iPhones and apps, he used the recorder to capture key meetings or random action items and thoughts. The tape still inside contained a recording of the two of us negotiating a licensing deal for the company that we worked for when we first met. Most of it was mind-numbingly dull, but every few minutes, I heard him interject a clever point or ask a thoughtful question that reminded me of a different life. I packed items away in his closet, ready to move them but not to be rid of them.

I started with one dresser, then the other, and then the bathroom vanity. Once I finished the bedroom, I tackled the garage. Project after project, I transformed the house until it felt like mine. So much of him was still there, but I selected the good and packed away the bad. I realized I could keep living in our house, a concept I was unsure of in the beginning. With spaces reclaimed and everything in order, I actually wanted to live in the house. It reminded me of Russ, and he was such a big part of me. I couldn't imagine letting it go.

Unfortunately, there were only so many closets and rooms to organize. I'd stepped away from my job to care for Russ, and the unknown for the next phase of my life started to plague me. As I sat home in the quiet with the kids at school and no job to go to, I looked around. For the first time since I was nineteen years old, I didn't have a boyfriend or a husband as a constant companion. It was only me. Well, me and two little humans who watched my every move.

I repeated the same questions over and over again. Who am I? Who do I want to be? It became clear that I wasn't sure.

I'd already fielded calls from colleagues offering opportunities. Some were for consulting, and some were for full-time gigs. As they described the fabulous little widget that promised to revolutionize the world, the voice in my head that used to latch on and engage instead sat back and said, "Meh." I couldn't go back to the grind of someone else's vision. I wanted to create my own vision and start or join something that furthered it. But what the hell was my vision?

I started with the basics. Forget vision; I needed to get clear on values. What values were most important to me? I scribbled and erased and scribbled again, and after a few days, I came up with six core values that now grace the wall of my kitchen.

Number one: Health. I understand my body, mind, and spirit, and I prioritize the things that keep them strong. My journey showed me that without health, there was nothing else. It was the top, the pinnacle, the most important. And that didn't only mean exercising and eating right. They were essential, but it was also vital to listen to my body. I no longer accepted bloating or crankiness. I figured out what I ate that caused it and avoided that food. I recognized when I felt anxious or fearful, and I stopped and meditated to change my mindset. It wasn't okay to be out of shape, and it wasn't okay to be depressed. My body and mind were telling me something, and I needed to slow down and listen.

Number Two: Family. I embrace my family as my core, my rock, and my center. Those two little kids, my two crazy dogs, my parents, my brother—they were everything. In whatever I did next, I couldn't lose sight of that massive truth.

Number Three: Growth. I learn and experience every day and use the knowledge I gain as a beacon for others. Learning made me happy. It kept my brain healthy. My tragedy exposed me to fascinating advances in science that would become the future of medicine. I hungered to learn more, and I longed to bring that future to the present.

Number Four: Friends. I surround myself with amazing people, and I treat my good friends like family. Russ's disease was isolating. I craved the love and laughter of my friends. In my brief time back in the world, I'd reconnected with so many fabulous people. That tribe was a crucial part of keeping me whole.

Number Five: Independence. I cultivate the habits and routines that make me financially and emotionally independent. Russ and I had worked hard all of our lives. That hard work left me blessed with financial freedom and the opportunity to take time to heal. I realized that most people didn't live that way. My kids lived in a big house and didn't want for much. I needed to ensure they had the tools to grow independent. I wanted them to live within their means and be happy in the process. Happy—that part was critical. I'd spent too much time letting the emotions of others dictate my mood and my feelings. I needed to take control and find happiness within.

Number Six: Fun. I seek fun and enjoyment in everything that I do. Russ had excelled at bringing joy into our lives. I'd always envied his humor and how he made everyone around him laugh. His disease surgically removed that from my house, and I wanted it back. I wanted my home to be a place to gather, a place of laughter, a place of warm memories.

There they were, the first-ever Bell Family Values. I didn't know where they would lead, but I knew if I held to them, I'd be proud of whatever happened.

But while I strove to rebuild, Russ continued to decline. His descent was not a straight line, but a series of steep plunges that stabilized for indeterminate periods of time. It was like a blind descent down stairs of arbitrary size. Two and a half years after placing him in Brookhaven, he was finally at peace. After over five years of torment, I expected his passing to bring mostly relief. Instead, it was like losing him all over again.

But by that point, I'd worked myself up to a big decision—it was time to start dating again. I never intended that milestone to coincide with his death, but my self-imposed deadline, set months before, ended up being within thirty days of his passing. It made initial interactions interesting.

"Oh, you're a widow? I'm so sorry. When did your husband pass?"

"Well, actually, it was last month." The factual statement felt false since I'd lost him years before and brought a series of eyebrow raises from potential dates.

But I persisted through the awkwardness, unsure what I'd find. I tempered my expectations after hearing years of dating horror stories from divorced friends. Plus, Russ was my soul mate.

Did a person get more than one? It seemed unlikely, particularly now that I was in my mid-forties, had two kids, and was definitely set in my ways.

I settled into a convenient relationship that was fun but not right, and convinced myself that it was enough. I was enough, so having someone who filled in little holes and voids was all I needed.

And then I met Keith.

Keith introduced himself while we were waiting to watch our sons play baseball. I had noticed him before and knew he looked familiar, but I couldn't figure out why. He had the same feeling and decided to say hello. As it turned out, we both worked in medical devices and had several common connections. We swapped numbers and agreed to have lunch.

I soon knew that he was meant for me. It was like I'd subconsciously written a job description for the perfect partner, and then God or karma or whatever rules the earth delivered him directly to my folding chair. I felt fortunate, loved, and happy, but I also felt something else rise from the ashes—fear.

I searched my emotions for the source of this unwanted guest. It wasn't fear of being hurt by Keith. He made me feel safe and loved in a way I'd never experienced, even when Russ was well. And it wasn't fear of Russ's disapproval. Unlike other widows I'd talked to, I'd never received the "I want you to find someone and be happy" speech from Russ. It was quite the opposite. His diseased, anxious mind was paranoid about losing me, and he often accused me of having an affair when I was away from Brookhaven. But I knew the man I married thought differently. He would have handled the situation in the same way I handled Daisy. He would want me and the kids to be happy. Fear of Russ's disapproval wasn't it.

So what was it? Then, I noticed when my fear peaked. Every minor complaint of spurious pain or emotion from Keith sent me reeling. I'd contemplate, analyze, and wonder; that cycle unearthed the root. My fear was that Keith would die too. I feared that some horrible disease would enter our world and throw me back into the abyss of caregiving. That the support and comfort I was just getting used to would be ripped away, and my feet, now solid and grounded, would hurl back on a slippery slope of ice.

The subconscious worry plagued my thoughts, but the conscious acknowledgement of my fear held no relief. Life ends with death, for some, sooner than others. Dealing with death wasn't just possible; it was inevitable. The only variables were order and timing. And with my history, all that left was worry.

But a dear friend once advised me to reframe worry. Worry is frenetic, useless energy that leads nowhere. It lacks productivity and purpose. Instead, he suggested that I reframe worry into awareness. I'm aware that Keith may become ill and die. The same is true for me. With that awareness, we can take action. We can engage in preventative medicine and screen for key markers of disease. We can ensure that we eat well, exercise, and listen to our bodies. We can use what I've learned in my experience with Russ to monitor for signs and symptoms in a way that is action-oriented and helpful. It may not avert disaster, but I'm also aware that this disaster may never come.

So I move on. I acknowledge my loss and fear and reframe it. Caregiving is hard, and the work doesn't end with the assignment. There are scars, some superficial and some deep. They linger and rear their heads in places they don't seem to belong until I unpack the reasons behind their presence.

But my caregiving journey has left me stronger and more resilient. I'm rebuilding myself, but not into what I was—that would be impossible. Instead, I'm rebuilding myself into someone more thoughtful, more compassionate, and more grateful. That is the cosmic gift that comes to balance what feels like unending caregiving hell. When living in that hell, I would never have believed it. But now, from the other side, I know that by hanging in and doing the work, that gift was destined to come.

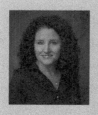

Nicole Bell is a mom and successful entrepreneur. As an executive in a fast-growing medical device company, she built a world-class team in surgical robotics. In 2017, Nicole's husband was diagnosed with a devastating disease, and she was forced into her most challenging roles yet: caregiver and medical proxy. Unsatisfied with the doctors' answers, Nicole used her engineering mindset to search for the root causes of her husband's illness. She eventually found them and sought treatment—a process that changed her entire view of modern medicine.

Nicole grew up near Boston, earned a Bachelor's and Master's of Science in Materials Science and Engineering from MIT and a Master's of Science in Biomedical Engineering from Duke University. She currently lives near Raleigh, North Carolina, with her two children and dogs. For more information on Nicole, please visit www.nicoledaniellebell.com.

EPILOGUE

Our oldest former US President, Jimmy Carter, decided to forego treatment of his cancer in favor of hospice care at home, surrounded by family and friends. It's a common phrase used in obituaries, *surrounded by family and friends*, but how often do we think about the distinction between the two groups?

In simple terms, family members are those who share our DNA or join the family through adoption or marriage. Friends are people who enter your life through shared experiences, common interests, or needs. If you are lucky, the line between these two groups becomes blurred, so you can't tell one from the other.

At the beginning of your caregiving journey, friends and family become the bedrock of your support system. These are the people you turn to, rely on, and need in order to function properly and provide care for your loved one. Over time, you may see some of that initial support subside, but don't let that discourage you from asking for help.

Mike Tenaglia has been on his caregiving journey for more than ten years. In his experience, some family members will disappoint you, and some friends will rise up and support you in every meaningful way. Mike told me about his youth, growing up in a small village in Italy. Sometimes, the only way to survive was to rely on your neighbors. He lives on Cape Cod now, yet he still relies on neighbors for help, depending on Lynda's health and treatment schedule. Each time he asks for help, it is met with an enthusiastic and affirmative response. They never ask him for anything in return because they know when the time comes, he will return the favor without hesitation.

Alan Rubel's cancer caregiving journey lasted thirteen years. Regrettably, his wife, Sharon, succumbed to the dreadful disease four years ago. Alan found out that support and help aren't limited by geographic boundaries. He and Mike Tenaglia met in the waiting room while their wives were in the recovery at Mass General Brigham. They have been close friends since, providing much-needed encouragement and support to one another, despite the more than three hours of driving distance between them.

In fact, it's why you just finished reading this book. The two friends wanted to share a common message of hope, humility, and love to caregivers throughout the world. I believe they have achieved that goal, for throughout *The Greatest Burden The Greatest Blessing* are amazing stories of courage, strength, and love.

Yet you also read about one of the most difficult parts of being a caregiver—*care for the caregiver*. How much stress, loneliness, fear, anxiety, mental and physical pain, and, in some cases, financial burden, can we endure?

As it turns out, more than we realize—but with some asterisks.

Neglecting your own personal care will undoubtedly impact the care you give to your loved one. The challenge for many isn't going to be *will you ask for help*, but likely, *will you accept help?* Why? Because we're stubborn and we don't want to impose upon people. Yet, more often than not, people want to help us.

Here are some suggestions to keep in mind when considering your own care:

*Ask for help—or accept it when offered. No matter how big or small, accept the help. And when it arrives, do something for yourself without an ounce of guilt.

*Don't skip out on your own medical appointments and checkups. Find ways to include moderate exercise in your day, and don't abandon healthy eating habits. Just because you're in this role doesn't mean you can eat as much junk food as you want. Without the proper hydration and nutrition, you are even more prone to sickness, whether it be a common cold or something more serious.

*Join a support group, find a caregiving program, or seek therapy for yourself. If possible, don't wait until the burdens of caregiving are too heavy. If you can't speak to someone, writing down your thoughts in a journal can be very helpful.

*Don't ignore invitations to be social with your friends—your loved one wouldn't like that, and it's definitely not good for your long-term mental health. Maybe find a new hobby or return to an old one. There's only so much stress you can handle, and these activities are crucial in order to rest your brain, body, and spirit.

*If you're able to, consider hiring part-time help to give you a break during the week or weekend. Maybe there's a teenager in your area who can sit with your care recipient for an hour. Or ask a neighbor, relative, or friend to do the same.

*Get enough sleep, or I should say, take it when you can get it. Sleep deprivation can lead to poor decision-making, and you need to be mentally and physically sharp in your caregiving role.

Having cared for my dad with Alzheimer's, I know these suggestions can be anything but simple, so don't beat yourself up if you feel that one or more of them begin to slip. Just do your best to make a consistent effort to follow them.

But here's the other side of the caregiving coin: it's an opportunity to hit the reset button.

The reality is, most of us wait for tragedy to strike before realizing that we need to change. Whether that change is related to our health, mindset, relationships, or career—we don't have to wait for a life-altering event in order to change the narrative of our life's story. None of us are obligated to be the person we were forty years ago, fourteen years ago, four years ago, or four weeks ago.

My father's Alzheimer's was anything but a blessing, but caring for him was. I got to know him better than at any point in my life, and it was during my caregiving journey that my perspective and outlook on life changed. I was able to let go of past regrets and grudges and excuses for my short-comings; I was able to appreciate and understand how fragile life is and finally accept that we all have demons, flaws, and limitations. But none of them need to define who we are or who we want to be.

If there was a magic cure for Alzheimer's and he were still alive today, I wouldn't need his thanks for taking care of him during his time of greatest need—but he would give it to me anyway. In reply, I would tell my dad that I would do it all over again, without hesitation, because there's almost nothing we can't handle in the name of love.

We don't always know the outcome when we answer the call to serve as a caregiver, yet we answer it anyway. Some of us don't get to experience a happy ending, but that doesn't mean our caregiving duties were for nothing. Don't ever doubt your impact as a caregiver. The unconditional love you provided in that role was most definitely felt, appreciated, and cherished by the recipient. Although they may not have been able to express their gratitude, there's no doubt in my mind that they will find a way to make it known.

I thought an appropriate way to end *The Greatest Burden The Greatest Blessing* was to hear directly from some of the care recipients written about in the book. Their lives were forever changed by devastating injuries, addiction, and diseases—yet even more so by those who mended, supported, and cared for them—thus, receiving the greatest blessing imaginable: love.

Thank you for being part of our journey.

Mark J. Resnick

P.S. If you'd like to help others discover our book, please take a minute to write a review of our book on Amazon. It can be one line or a few sentences, but it would mean a lot to us to receive your honest feedback.

Go to: www.caregivingguys.com/review.

BOB HALLORAN

Care recipient of Eileen Curran.

Her story is found on page 65

Dear Eileen:

During the more than 20 years you and I have been together, I have watched with awe as you have given so much of your time, energy, and talents to help others. You are, without question, the most compassionate and generous person I know. So, it came as no surprise when you came through for me in such a big and loving way. Thank you! And in case I haven't said it enough – thank you, thank you, thank you, I love you!

You and I have talked about how, as a reporter covering tragic and sorrowful events, you had to compartmentalize your emotions and focus on telling the story. It's a learned and necessary skill, and I know you utilized that superpower in the weeks and months following my ruptured brain aneurysm. I also know you worried about me, and feared our children might lose their father, but you kept it together, and kept our family together through one of our most difficult times.

We've also talked about how I was a bit of an ogre in the hospital. I'm still sorry about that, and again, I thank you for not holding that against me, and for loving the worst of me. I will forever be equal parts lucky to have you, and grateful for all the things you did, and continue to do for me.

Love always,
Me

P.S. Thank you, thank you, thank you, I love you!

KELLY DEVITT

Care recipient of Ed Devitt.

His story is found on page 15

I don't know if it's possible to express my appreciation for the team of caregivers who kept me alive, and then allowed me to have a life after my accident. I thank the Lord first, for his blessings, then Janice and Cecilia, my current caregivers. And, of course you, Dad. The only way to say this, Dad, is I have unending gratitude for you.

God Bless everyone who has experienced a traumatic brain injury.

-Kelly

LESLIE COHEN

Care recipient of Joyce Khan.
Her story is found on page 21

I love my sister, but for quite a long time before I became ill, I had been ambivalent about her. I adored her as a child, but her jealousy manifested in all sorts of unpleasant ways and kept coming between us. And while I empathized with her feelings of low self-esteem, over time, after various incidents, I simply closed down around her and vowed not to open myself again to the hurt. Until I got sick. With the very strong encouragement of our brother, I accepted Joyce's offer to help me during my recovery. I wasn't sure what kind of caregiver she would be. I was always the family caregiver, and I knew I would not be in a position to take care of her.

But Joyce not only rose to the occasion—she soared. She put herself in situations that were extremely challenging, like helping with frightening-looking wounds, giving infusions, making food I could swallow, driving on heavily-trafficked roads to take me to medical appointments more than an hour away, and a whole lot more, which she did with grace and graciousness. Most importantly, though, she was there, and it was incredibly reassuring and comforting simply to have her there with me. We "bonded," grabbed the opportunity of time together, put the past behind, and became both friends and sisters again.

I am eternally grateful.
-Leslie

PHIL DOHERTY

Care recipient of Julie Doherty.

Her story is found on page 141

I don't remember putting my boots on that day. I certainly didn't see the crane heading my way, but I definitely heard my body crunch and felt immeasurable pain upon impact. I was conscious and spitting up blood. A colleague was rubbing my legs. "Don't tell Julie," I told him before the EMT arrived, but I knew he had to.

I flatlined on the way to the hospital. I saw clouds in the distance—or, more accurately, I looked directly into a large, oval-shaped, white cloud. I spoke to my youngest son, Colin, and told him, "Be good to your mom." The only other memories of my first two weeks in a coma were the dreams. Especially the one where I was on a dock, hanging on a hook like a giant fish. My chest cavity was wide open, and they were rinsing out my insides. All the blood flowed in the ocean. Like they had to wash me out.

An incredible team of doctors, nurses, therapists—and many other unseen individuals who work in these facilities—put me back together. They allowed me to live, but it was Julie who saved my life. She made the important decisions, the ones that were going to make or break my chances of surviving the accident. Once it became apparent that I would survive, none of us were sure I would ever walk again.

Six days a week, she was by my side. Julie took Sundays off because in her words, "There was too much traffic on Sundays to go into Boston!" We joked about it, but she needed that day off. She was so emotionally and physically drained.

My rehabilitation was supposed to be six months, but I was home two weeks later. I was determined—no, more like obsessed—to return to work within a year. Most people thought I was nuts. My doctors did. But Julie was thrilled. She knew that's how I was wired and encouraged me every step of the way. There's no way I would have met that goal without her support.

I got lucky; I really did. Almost everything went right for me. Our families stepped up big time to assist Julie and friends did the same. My boss, Gus Delfarno, visited me every day in the hospital and was a huge help to Julie. My brother and sister-in-law were so incredible as well. I will never be able to properly thank them.

But Julie—you were the one who saved my life. I've loved you since we were seventeen and will always love you. Thank you for saving my life and our family.

-Phil

BRIAN GREENBLOTT

Care recipient of Art and Ginny Greenblott.
Their story is found on page 223

I'm approaching twenty-two years of sobriety and what a long journey it has been. I consider myself one of the lucky ones, in that it worked out for me. What people don't often understand is that addiction is a family illness. It's not just the addict that suffers and spirals downward. Addiction brings the entire family down, and when the addict doesn't get better, the families remain sick, too. Without the family's support, education, and commitment to a process of recovery for the addict, it's very hard, if not impossible, for the addict to recover—or stay alive.

Mom, Dad, Kara, Kevin, and Lisa—thank you for never giving up on me. Thank you for never giving up hope that one day I could overcome my demons and addiction. You stepped up to the plate and educated yourselves about the disease, attended recovery meetings, and made the difficult decision to draw the line in the sand by telling me, "We love you, Brian, but if you're not going to get better—we are."And that's why my recovery happened.

To Michael Herbert—I owe you my life. Without your intervention, encouragement, and steadfast belief in me, I'd be dead. It's because of you that my family never gave up on me and committed to healing themselves, which then allowed me to recover. And you're the reason why I started Reco Intensive, so that others suffering from chemical dependence could renew their commitment to sobriety and restore their capacity for healing.

I hope this book and the stories within it give hope to those suffering from addiction, disease, and injury. For individuals and families afflicted by addiction, I am always available. You can reach me at bgreenblott@recointensive.com.

TIM KAVANAGH

Care recipient of Candy Kavanagh.
Her story is found on page 55

Candy and I had been dating for nine months back in 2016. Then the stage II colorectal cancer diagnosis came. At the time, I thought, "Well, that was fun!" She was a single Mom to two teenagers and owned her own business. There's no way she's going to want any part of this—the relationship or potential caregiving role.

But Candy and I shared a very powerful bond from the beginning, and our love for one another grows stronger each day. She's my true soulmate in life, and I count my blessings every day.

Since the diagnosis in 2016, Candy has been with me every step of the way. And because Candy loves so fiercely, she is the ultimate caregiver. From the beginning, I've been in awe of her presence and patience; her strength and courage. I remember shortly after the diagnosis when I was approved for a clinical trial. They handed us this giant three-ring binder full of information. Our nurse went through that binder page by page. My mind was numb to almost everything, but Candy listened, took notes, asked questions, researched on her own, and was a key part of every decision made regarding my health—then and now.

Then, there was the time the hospital staff wanted to discharge me without a solution to my complications from the temporary ileostomy I received as part of my sectioning surgery. We had just gone through a sleepless weekend of hell with the bag not being able to stay on for more than 20 minutes. The four bags of supplies that Candy commandeered with the nurse before we left were all but gone! When the surgeon and wound care team said there was nothing more they could do, Candy stood up and went through the weekend's events. She told them flat out that they WOULD find a bed and that they WOULD tend to the wounds until a solution was found. I like to think of this as one of Candy's mild Shirley McClaine moments from 'Terms of Endearment'.

Whether it's my personal or medical care, my emotional state of mind, or stepping in to take over everything related to household responsibilities, I could not be in better hands or with a better partner than Candy. I'm so grateful and blessed to have a caregiver and spouse like her. I know not everyone is so lucky.

That's why I think this book is so important—because the dedication, compassion, and commitment caregivers display each and every day is extraordinary. PLEASE recognize a caregiver that you know and thank them. Let them know the important work that they do for the person(s) they are caring for. Overall, caregivers play a vital role in enhancing the quality of life for individuals who require assistance. Their dedication, compassion, and commitment make a significant difference in the lives of those they support, enabling them to maintain dignity, independence, and a sense of belonging within their communities.

Candy Cane, I would be lost without you. Everything you do for me, for us, and our families is so remarkable that it's hard for me to capture in words. Thank you for being my caregiver, advocate, best friend, and soulmate.

E2E, L2L, H2H, S2S

-Tim

ACKNOWLEDGEMENTS

It started in a waiting room at Massachusetts General Brigham Hospital. Alan Rubel and I sat across from each other, waiting for our spouses, Sharon and Lynda, who were both recovering from surgical procedures in their respective battles against cancer. Then we met again later, this time in the recovery room. Some may call it coincidence—others may call it destiny.

The conversations that followed the encounters left a profound impact on both of us. From favorite Boston restaurants to sports, cancer, and caregiving, Alan and I agreed to keep in touch. And we did. These two caregiving guys became great friends and relied upon each other for support, encouragement, and kinship.

After Sharon passed, we remained close, and together, we planted the seeds for *The Greatest Burden The Greatest Blessing*. Mark Resnick became the third caregiving guy not long after his caregiving memoir, *Ten Days With Dad*, was published. Mark's been the foundation for our endeavor; without him, I'm not sure this book would have come to fruition. I speak for Alan in expressing our eternal gratitude for his talent and friendship.

But none of this would be possible were it not for the misfortune and remarkable strength of my beautiful wife, Lynda. She has been fighting cancer for more than ten years—since that fateful day, February 5, 2013. I am grateful she has allowed me to be by her side during this most difficult time in our lives. Each day has been a struggle, yet when the opportunity presents itself, we try to escape reality with short trips to New York for a play or Bermuda for some sunshine. While these getaways have offered glimpses of a normal life, cancer is always there to remind us of our reality and the disease. Still, I am grateful that I could provide Lynda with those brief respites from cancer.

I want to thank my daughter, Maria, son-in-law, Aaron, and grandchildren, Abby and Jack. They provide times of calmness and distraction when

Lynda needs relief from the disease. I am thankful to my brother for his daily phone calls to check on Lynda and invitations to meet for coffee or lunch. These types of outreaches are what caregivers need—normal interactions— to distract us from the constant state of stress and anxiety.

I would also like to acknowledge my friends and colleagues who gave me the latitude to make plans and break them because Lynda needed me more. But they kept asking and accommodated my needs, and I am grateful.

To the countless patients and caregivers I have met over the years, your strength, courage, and perseverance have truly been an inspiration and given me the strength to persevere in my own continued support of Lynda.

There are many more who deserve thanks and gratitude, some of whom don't even know they did anything to help. They don't realize that the simple phone call, text, note, and words of encouragement mean so much to Lynda and me.

Most of all, I need to thank Lynda for being so strong in her fight and showing me that together, anything can be accomplished, even fighting cancer.

-Michael D. Tenaglia

***

To Sharon, my loving partner who has passed—a loving daughter, sister, mother, grandmother, and friend to all, who encouraged me to write this book for caregivers and caregivers-to-be.

To Robert and Jill, and my grandchildren, Cole and Lucy, for all their support and help.

To Heather, for her continued love and support. ♥

To Cornelius "Con" Hogan, whose wisdom and inspiration motivated me to move forward with the writing of this book.

To my fellow caregiver guys, Mike Tenaglia and Mark Resnick. I want to thank them for their generosity, talents, and passion. Making this amazing book with them was a true blessing.

To our story writers/caregivers who contributed to our fantastic book, may the Greatest Blessing be with you and your families.

-Alan E. Rubel

***

After publishing my first book, *Ten Days With Dad,* in 2022, the plan was to promote the book for two years and then begin another one. That plan changed less than six months later when Alan Rubel and Mike Tenaglia invited me to co-author *The Greatest Burden The Greatest Blessing*. These two guys have inspired me every day since, and I'm so grateful for that invitation, their trust, and our friendship.

Coleen and I have been walking together since 1992. It started at Campion Hall, and I have no intention of thinking about when it might end. Thank you, Col, for supporting my every step, stumble, and, yes, crash! You're always there to pick me up, steady me—and keep me moving forward. Thank you *maui* much. Always.

To Campbell, Erin, and Sean, nothing makes me prouder than you three. And remember—own your story, pursue your passion, and love yourself.

To the caregivers who let me share their stories for this book, thank you. It was a privilege I will never forget.

Big D, Mo, AA, Aunt Linda—and the rest of my angels—thanks for lifting me up when I need it most.

-Mark J. Resnick

RESOURCES

The following list of resources is meant to serve as a starting point in your caregiving journey. While online resources are the most abundant, you will find excellent resources in your local library as well. Perhaps the best way to find more information on a particular health topic is by asking someone you know and trust who has already been through the experience.

For more information and expanded resources, visit www.caregivingguys.com.

Addiction

Substance Abuse and Mental Health Services Administration

www.samhsa.gov

Alcoholics Anonymous

www.aa.org

Drug Abuse Foundation

www.dafpbci.org

Reco Intensive

www.recointensive.com

Alzheimer's

Alzheimer's Association

www.alz.org

Alzheimer's.gov

www.alzheimers.gov

AlzAuthors

www.alzauthors.com

Autism

Autism Partnership Foundation

www.autism-foundation.org

Autism Speaks

www.autismspeaks.org

ABA Centers of America

www.abacenters.com

Cancer

National Cancer Institute Live Help

https://livehelp.cancer.gov/app/chat/chat_launch

National Cancer Institute

www.cancer.gov

American Cancer Society

www.cancer.org

Cancer Support Community

www.cancersupportcommunity.org

Mass General Brigham Cancer Center

https://because.massgeneral.org/caregivingresearch

Caregiving

National Institute on Aging

www.nia.nih.gov

Three Things Thursday *on caregiving

www.threethingthursday.com/newsletter

Daily Caring

www.dailycaring.com

Downs syndrome

Downs Syndrome Resource Foundation

www.dsrf.org

<h1 style="text-align:center">Hospice</h1>

National Association for Home Care & Hospice

https://community.nahc.org/home

<h1 style="text-align:center">Lyme Disease</h1>

Lyme Disease Foundation

www.lyme.org

<h1 style="text-align:center">Mental Health</h1>

American Foundation for Suicide Prevention

https://afsp.org

National Institute on Mental Health

www.nimh.nih.gov

<h1 style="text-align:center">Parkinson's</h1>

Parkinson's Foundation

www.parkinson.org

Davis Phinney Foundation

www.davisphinneyfoundation.org

Michael J. Fox Foundation

www.michaeljfox.org

110 Fitness

www.110fitness.org

<h1 style="text-align:center">PTSD/Veteran's Care</h1>

Veterans Affairs

www.va.gov

HOW CAN YOU HELP?

Enjoy the book?

Here are three ways to help us get the book into the hands of more readers.

1. Take a minute to write a review of our book on Amazon. It can be one line or a few sentences, but it would mean a lot to receive your honest feedback. Log in to your Amazon account and find your purchase, or go to www.caregivingguys.com/review to be taken directly to your login, the review page.

2. Share the book with friends and family on social media. Use #greatestblessingbook or share our website with them: www.caregivingguys.com

3. Donate a copy to your local library, assisted/independent living community, nursing home or nonprofit. Use coupon code DONATE at checkout from our website, and you will receive $5 off your total purchase.

4. If you would like to share your story for the next edition of *The Greatest Burden The Greatest Blessing*, go to www.caregivingguys.com/share-your-story.

Thank you!

BOOK SPONSORS

VIP SPONSOR

Brian Greenblott is an addict, one who has been clean and sober going on 26 years. His parents, Arthur and Ginny, shared their story for the book, which can be found on page 223.

Brian is the co-owner of RECO Intensive in Delray Beach, FL. RECO's mission serves to restore light and color to the lives of those suffering from addiction. Through their experiential and comprehensive treatment solutions, they aim to provide a secure, respectful, and empathetic environment in which individuals can truly recover.

Visit www.recointensive.com to get started on your recovery.

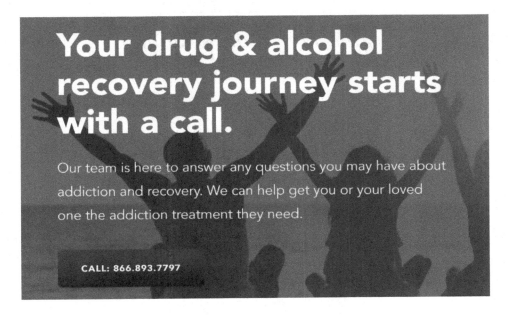

Your drug & alcohol recovery journey starts with a call.

Our team is here to answer any questions you may have about addiction and recovery. We can help get you or your loved one the addiction treatment they need.

CALL: 866.893.7797

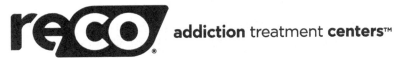

reco addiction treatment centers™

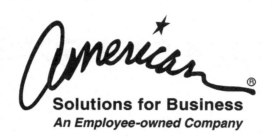

Solutions for Business

An Employee-owned Company

BELCHER FITZGERALD LLP

COUNSELLORS AT LAW

BUSINESS • LITIGATION • TRUSTS & ESTATES

www.belcherfitzgerald.com

The Campbells

Jim, Tim, Dan, & John

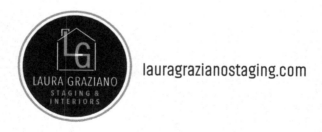

lauragrazianostaging.com

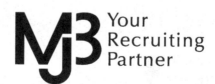

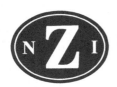 **NAMAKSY-ZAMMITO INSURANCE AGENCY, INC.**
nziagency.com

 NORTHEAST PLANNING ASSOCIATES, INC.
A Registered Investment Adviser

FRICKE FINANCIAL
www.frickefinancial.com

John F. Fricke, CLU, ChFC
(802) 485-6953
john.fricke@lpl.com

Thomas W. Fricke, CRPC®
(802) 778-0545
thomas.fricke@lpl.com

Securities offered through LPL Financial, member FINRA/SIPC. Northeast Planning
Associates, Inc. and Fricke Financial are separate entities from LPL Financial.

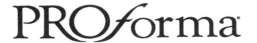

RUSS HOWARTH

CHARLES JANOSIC

ANDREW JANOSIC

ROSS LEVINE

KEVIN MONTECALVO

KEVIN AND MARY LOU O'CONNOR

JEFF ROTHCHILD

JAY VENTO

Spruce Mountain Granites &
Custom Sandblast, Inc.

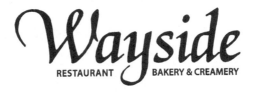

BARRE VT LIONS CLUB

BARRE VT ROTARY

Dr. William Koch, DDS

EDDIE ROUSSE LIFE INSURANCE AGENCY

Joshua Singer, L.Ac. ACUPUNCTURE

Scott Cameron

Rob Carr, CAPITOL STEEL & SUPPLY COMPANY

CHASE & CHASE LAND SURVEYOR

CLINTON SAVINGS BANK, www.clintonsavings.com

Bob Cody, CODY CHEVROLET, Montpelier, VT

Fredda Fox Stimell

John Gardner, GARDNER INSURANCE SERVICES INC

Ginny and Arthur Greenblott

J A GOULD PLUMBING & HEATING INC

Matt Grundy, BUILDER SPECIALTIES INC.

HOOKER AND WHITCOMB FUNERAL HOME

Vicki Langevin

Tomas Lauzon, ACCOUNTANT

LENNY'S SHOE & APPAREL

Craig Martin & COHASSET INSURANCE

Matthew Peterson, UPWARD MOBILITIY

MORRISON & CLARK CARPET, INC.

MORSE FARM MAPLE SUGARWORKS

NEWFIELD HOUSE, www.newfieldhouse.com

ORMSBY'S COMPUTER SYSTEMS

PHOENIX BOOKS, Burlington, VT

PRUNEAU-POLLI FUNERAL HOME

Nathan Royea, VERMONT DOOR COMPANY

John Scheer, SCHEER & HICKEY, PC ACCOUNTING FIRM

Mark Tatro, TATRO APPLIANCE

Jill and Robert Vandor

Laynie and David Vandor

VFW Post 790, Barre, VT

110 Fitness, Rockland, MA

Josh Peach – Be Au Sm

Candy Nelson Cavanagh

Janet Steward